SpringerBriefs in Psy

SpringerBriefs present concise summaries of cutting-edge research and practical applications across a wide spectrum of fields. Featuring compact volumes of 50 to 125 pages, the series covers a range of content from professional to academic. Typical topics might include:

- A timely report of state-of-the-art analytical techniques
- A bridge between new research results as published in journal articles and a contextual literature review
- A snapshot of a hot or emerging topic
- An in-depth case study or clinical example
- A presentation of core concepts that readers must understand to make independent contributions

SpringerBriefs in Psychology showcase emerging theory, empirical research, and practical application in a wide variety of topics in psychology and related fields. Briefs are characterized by fast, global electronic dissemination, standard publishing contracts, standardized manuscript preparation and formatting guidelines, and expedited production schedules.

More information about this series at http://www.springer.com/series/10143

Victor Counted • Richard G. Cowden
Haywantee Ramkissoon

Place and Post-Pandemic Flourishing

Disruption, Adjustment, and Healthy Behaviors

☘ Springer

Victor Counted
School of Psychology
Western Sydney University
Penrith, NSW, Australia

Richard G. Cowden
Human Flourishing Program, Institute for Quantitative Social Science
Harvard University
Cambridge, MA, USA

Haywantee Ramkissoon
College of Business, Law & Social Sciences
Derby Business School, University of Derby
Derby, UK

ISSN 2192-8363 ISSN 2192-8371 (electronic)
SpringerBriefs in Psychology
ISBN 978-3-030-82579-9 ISBN 978-3-030-82580-5 (eBook)
https://doi.org/10.1007/978-3-030-82580-5

© The Author(s), under exclusive licence to Springer Nature Switzerland AG 2021
This work is subject to copyright. All rights are solely and exclusively licensed by the Publisher, whether the whole or part of the material is concerned, specifically the rights of translation, reprinting, reuse of illustrations, recitation, broadcasting, reproduction on microfilms or in any other physical way, and transmission or information storage and retrieval, electronic adaptation, computer software, or by similar or dissimilar methodology now known or hereafter developed.
The use of general descriptive names, registered names, trademarks, service marks, etc. in this publication does not imply, even in the absence of a specific statement, that such names are exempt from the relevant protective laws and regulations and therefore free for general use.
The publisher, the authors, and the editors are safe to assume that the advice and information in this book are believed to be true and accurate at the date of publication. Neither the publisher nor the authors or the editors give a warranty, expressed or implied, with respect to the material contained herein or for any errors or omissions that may have been made. The publisher remains neutral with regard to jurisdictional claims in published maps and institutional affiliations.

This Springer imprint is published by the registered company Springer Nature Switzerland AG
The registered company address is: Gewerbestrasse 11, 6330 Cham, Switzerland

This book is dedicated to people all around the world whose connections to places of significance were disrupted due to the COVID-19 pandemic.

Contents

1	**Place Attachment During a Pandemic: An Introduction**	1
	Attachment Theory and Place: A Conceptual Clarification	2
	Multiple Domains of Place Attachment	3
	Emerging Place Dialectics During the COVID-19 Pandemic	4
	Emplacement–Displacement	4
	Inside–Outside	5
	Fixity–Flow	6
	Why Relationships with Place Matter in a Pandemic	7
	Structure of the Book	8
	References	9

Part I Place Attachment During a Pandemic

2	**Place Attachment During the COVID-19 Pandemic: A Scoping Review**	15
	Method	16
	Research Question	16
	Inclusion Criteria	16
	Literature Search	17
	Screening and Selection	17
	Data Extraction and Synthesis	19
	Results and Discussion	19
	Study Characteristics	19
	Summary of Findings	20
	Implications for Research and Practice	28
	Strengths and Limitations	30
	Conclusion	31
	References	31

3	**Place Attachment and Resource Loss During a Pandemic: An Ecological Systems Perspective**	33
	Conservation of Resources Theory and Principles	34
	Theory of Resource Loss	34
	Domains of Resource Loss	34
	Principles of Resource Loss	34
	Place Attachment Disruption and Resource Loss During the COVID-19 Pandemic: Separation from Significant Places and People in Place	37
	Place Attachment, Loss, and Recovery: Ecological Considerations During a Pandemic	38
	Ecological Propositions Associated with Place Attachment Disruption	41
	Proposition 1	41
	Proposition 2	41
	Proposition 3	41
	Proposition 4	42
	Conclusion	42
	References	43
4	**Place Attachment and Suffering During a Pandemic**	45
	Revisiting People-Place Relationships and Place Attachment Disruption	46
	Background on Suffering	47
	Place Attachment Disruption and Suffering	49
	Conclusion	51
	References	52
5	**Protest, Despair, and Detachment: Reparative Responses to Place Attachment Disruptions During a Pandemic**	55
	Background on Place Attachment Disruption	55
	Place Attachment Disruption During the COVID-19 Pandemic	57
	Disrupted Place Attachment at Multiple Spatial Domains During a Pandemic	58
	Reparative Responses to Place Attachment Disruption During a Pandemic	60
	Protest	60
	Despair	63
	Detachment	64
	Conclusion	66
	References	66

Part II Adjusting to Place Attachment Disruption During and After a Pandemic

6	**Adapting to Place Attachment Disruption During a Pandemic: From Resource Loss to Resilience**	71
	Psychological Distress of Place Attachment Disruption	72

	Rebounding from Resource Loss	73
	Mobilizing Religious/Spiritual Resources	74
	Building Religious/Spiritual Resources for Resilience	76
	Conclusion	77
	References	77
7	**Transcending Place Attachment Disruption: Strengthening Character During a Pandemic**	81
	Virtues and Character Strengths	82
	Pathways to Transcending Place Attachment Disruption: Gratitude, Hope, and Spirituality	83
	Gratitude	84
	Hope	85
	Spirituality	87
	Conclusion	88
	References	88
8	**Pro-environmental Behavior, Place Attachment, and Human Flourishing: Implications for Post-pandemic Research, Theory, Practice, and Policy**	93
	Pro-environmental Behavior as Planned Behavior	94
	From Pro-environmental Behavior to Place Attachment	95
	Place Attachment and Flourishing	97
	Fostering Place Flourishing After a Pandemic	99
	Identification	99
	Examination	100
	Design	100
	Evaluation	101
	Implications for Theory, Research, Policy, and Practice	102
	Theory	102
	Research	103
	Policy	104
	Practice	104
	Conclusion	105
	References	105
Index		109

Chapter 1
Place Attachment During a Pandemic: An Introduction

Victor Counted, Richard G. Cowden, and Haywantee Ramkissoon

Contents

Attachment Theory and Place: A Conceptual Clarification	2
Multiple Domains of Place Attachment	3
Emerging Place Dialectics During the COVID-19 Pandemic	4
Emplacement–Displacement	4
Inside–Outside	5
Fixity–Flow	6
Why Relationships with Place Matter in a Pandemic	7
Structure of the Book	8
References	9

The coronavirus disease 2019 (COVID-19) pandemic is an international health crisis. When the outbreak of severe acute respiratory syndrome coronavirus 2 (SARS-CoV-2) emerged, a lack of available treatment prompted widespread public health concerns (Govender et al., 2020). Countries and territories around the world implemented public health measures (e.g., stay-at-home orders, social distancing) to control the transmission of SARS-CoV-2 (Cowden et al., 2021). Non-essential travel and in-person social interactions were restricted. In several countries, educational institutions postponed in-person learning and places of worship were forced to substitute in-person services with online services. Employers also had to adapt to the legislative changes that were prompted by the public health crisis, with many reducing operations and requiring employees to work from home.

    The public health measures that were imposed in almost every part of the world forced people to change behavior patterns and reconfigure lifestyles to meet the public health and safety challenges of the COVID-19 pandemic (Counted et al., 2020). Although those measures were considered a necessary part of the public health response, an indirect consequence was that our interactions and bonds with significant places were disrupted. That disruption in people-place relationships has heightened our sense of awareness about the extent to which human life is inextricably tethered to places. It has also prompted us to more fully understand how the public health crisis has shifted people-place relationships, what our bonds with places might look like after the COVID-19 pandemic, and how connections between people and places can be restored and built again. Against the backdrop of the COVID-19 pandemic, this book discusses the implications of a public health crisis for our relationships with place. It also explores how society may recover and foster positive relations with places after a pandemic.

Attachment Theory and Place: A Conceptual Clarification

A useful framework for conceptualizing people-place relationships is attachment theory (Giuliani, 2003). Informed by the pioneering work of John Bowlby on attachment and loss, attachment experiences have been studied widely over the years. The attachment behavioral system develops during the early years of life through interactions with primary caregivers (Ainsworth, 1989; Bowlby, 1969). Attachment theory posits that caregivers, often in the form of a parent, caretaker, family member, or object, provide infants with a sense of physical comfort, security, and protection by being close in proximity. A caregiver functions as a secure base from which the infant explores the broader social environment. Research on attachment experiences has been extended to adults, with adult attachment theorists arguing that the mechanism of attachment is from *the cradle to the grave* because people grow into seeking substitute relationships with other objects of attachment later in life (Counted & Zock, 2019; Counted, 2018; Granqvist, 2020; Scannell & Gifford, 2014).

An object of attachment is anything that we invest emotional energy in. It can be transformed into a mental representation that influences our sense of self, others, and the world around us (Counted et al., 2021). Attachment objects can serve self-soothing functions during times of distress, provide a sense of felt security, and facilitate personal growth (Ainsworth, 1989; Bowlby, 1969). Adults usually have at least one meaningful object of attachment that they are connected to emotionally (Cicirelli, 1991, 2004).

Attachment experiences have been applied to people-place relationship experiences, with approximately three decades of empirical research published on place and attachment in environmental psychology (e.g., Lewicka, 2010; Low & Altman, 1992; Raymond et al., 2010; Scannell & Gifford, 2017). Research that intersects place and attachment theory falls under the umbrella theme of *place attachment*, which refers to the emotional bonds that people have with places of significance (Scannell & Gifford, 2010). Place attachment is one of the key research areas in environmental psychology that is used to examine human–environment interactions from a relational lens. From this perspective, *place* functions similarly to an internalized object or significant attachment object (Counted et al., 2021; Lewicka, 2011; Scannell & Gifford, 2010). It helps regulate difficult affective experiences (within the place domain), promotes identity development (within the process domain), and facilitates sociocultural meaning-making (within the person domain).

Place attachment overlaps conceptually with interpersonal attachment (Scannell & Gifford, 2014). Much like interpersonal attachment, place attachment helps people to regulate difficult emotional experiences and functions as a safe haven for those who have a sense of stability, security, rootedness, and comfort in a particular place (Relph, 1976; Scannell & Gifford, 2014). Place attachment also provides a *secure base* for those who identify with places (e.g., homes, places of worship, country) that form an important part of how they explore and relate to the broader environment. Similar to other objects of attachment, people can form a secure or insecure attachment with a place. For example, in the cases of domestic violence, childhood trauma, divorce, and places of trauma (e.g., 9/11 memorial site), ambivalence or negative attachment to place can develop (Manzo, 2003). A secure affective association with a place can help people to self-soothe, regulate self-esteem, and sustain connections to memories, history, ancestors, communal identity, and embodied spirituality (Captari et al., 2019; Counted et al., 2021; Sheldrake, 2019).

It follows then that separation distress is not only a response to separation or loss of an attachment figure, but it may also arise following a lost sense of connection to a place of significance (Bowlby, 1969; Scannell & Gifford, 2014). Separation distress may originate from a wide range of factors (e.g., natural disasters, pandemics, burglaries, voluntary relocations) and have adverse consequences (e.g., negative emotion, attachment insecurity) for people who have lost a sense of connection to a place of attachment (Marcheschi et al., 2015; Rollero & De Piccoli, 2010). Separation from a place of attachment can create a stressful period of *place attachment disruption* (Counted et al., 2021), which often triggers "a post-disruption phase of coping with lost attachments" (Brown & Perkins, 1992, p. 279). This experience occurs among migrants who must learn to adapt to a new environment and culture. That period of disruption usually leads to an outcome of positive adjustment characterized by attachment to the new environment (Ng, 1998).

Multiple Domains of Place Attachment

Place attachment is a multifaceted concept that intersects the affective, behavioral, and cognitive domains of place (Counted, 2016; Scannell & Gifford, 2010). These principal domains capture the interdependent contributions of people and the features of the environment to phenomenological experiences of place attachment (Scannell & Gifford, 2010; see also Counted et al., 2021; Jorgensen & Stedman, 2001; Lewicka, 2008). The *place* (or affective) domain entails attachment to the physical elements of a place (e.g., nature, architecture). Affective reactions to tangible physical attributes of place can include boredom, fear, excitement, and relaxation (Fornara et al., 2010). Some people may principally feel attached to the physical features of a place, such as the beauty of its scenery or the opportunities it presents for recreational activities (Lewicka, 2011). The *person* (or behavioral) domain emphasizes attachment to cultural and human lifeforms within a place (Seamon, 2012). Place attachment in this domain can happen through activities, milestones, memories, opportunities, or unique experiences one has in a particular place; social networks or interactions with people in a geographical space; or religious and cultural activities that make a place significant or meaningful.

The social dimension of place attachment has been studied extensively (Lewicka, 2011), given its role in fostering interpersonal relationships and sustaining group identity (Scannell & Gifford, 2010). Finally, the *process* (or cognitive) domain is where cultural and place identity are located. This domain addresses the association of place attachment with identity development and continuity. At its deepest level, place attachment supports character and identity formation within the context of place. Over time, the place of attachment becomes part of a person's self-concept and affects how they relate to themselves (Boğaç, 2009; Proshansky et al., 1983).

The trio of place attachment domains points to the salience of people-place relationships in human life. Threats to any of the domains can become a stressor or an obstacle to attachment. The COVID-19 pandemic has threatened each domain of place because it has affected our ability to access physical places (e.g., cities, workplaces, school campuses), restricted people from engaging in place-based activities (e.g., participating in events, interacting with friends or colleagues), and disrupted place identity. For example, we saw countries shut down their borders, in-person learning was suspended at schools, and many businesses had to close their doors. Each of those changes affected the place domain by limiting people from being able to access the physical spaces (e.g., school building, workplace) of places that are routinely part of their lives. The COVID-19 pandemic has shown how our relations with place can change, and it has brought about new place experiences as our interactions with familiar and favored places have become restricted. Maintaining the same quality of life in a particular place after a pandemic may be a serious challenge for those whose place attachments may have been disrupted by the pandemic.

Emerging Place Dialectics During the COVID-19 Pandemic

Three theoretical dialectics have been proposed to understand the impact of the COVID-19 pandemic on the relationships people have with places (Devine-Wright et al., 2020). These dialectics include emplacement–displacement, inside–outside, and fixity–flow. They each serve as a discourse between two different points of view about people-place relationships during the public health crisis. These dialectics are central to understanding the disruption of bonds that people have with places of significance. They also show how important it is for us to rethink the different and intricate meanings of people-place relationships within the context of a pandemic.

Emplacement–Displacement

The premise of the emplacement–displacement dialectic is that place is an ontological construction, and therefore our embodiment as human beings is embedded in place (Devine-Wright et al., 2020; Heidegger, 1958). This philosophical understanding intimates that human forms are shaped into *existence* and *being* within the context of place. In other words, life itself does not unfold outside of place. As humanity wrestles with concepts such as existence, being, becoming, and the nature of reality, the COVID-19 pandemic has amplified the importance of place as part of our ontological security[1] (Gustafsson & Krickel-Choi, 2020). More generally, the public health crisis has ushered in a new reality of an existence that involves being confined to our homes and emplacement experiences on a scale that is unprecedented.

The concept of emplacement is not only about being set in place. According to Devine-Wright et al. (2020), "it is an awareness of the tensions and nuances within [our] relationships [with place], and their impact on our ontological security" (p. 2). It is the *entrapping* and *stabilizing* experience of place in a pandemic situation. Turner (2010) described emplacement as a form of entrapment that is directly related to displacement during the COVID-19 pandemic. Public safety measures that emplace people may bring about experiences of displacement for those who are not adjusting well to pandemic-related challenges. Displacement within the context of the public health crisis underlies many of the ways that people have been separated from places that fulfill their needs. The COVID-19 pandemic has led to alienation from physical components of place, but people have also had their place-based memories and experiences disrupted (Honey-Rosés et al., 2020). Separation from places that form part of our everyday routines disrupts the bonds we have with places that hold significance in our lives, which can increase our vulnerability to the experience of displacement. The COVID-19 pandemic has highlighted the need to dedicate closer attention to the dialectical tension between emplacement and displacement.

Inside–Outside

The inside–outside dialectic moves away from understanding place as a bounded entity or a setting in which beings are embedded. Instead, it shows our interaction between *the inside and the outside* of a place (Kunstler, 1993). This interplay is what enables the individual to create meaning about a place through a constant comparison between what is inside versus outside, and in some cases will depend on one's access to what is outside. Curious exploration of the outside world is based on what is inside, as the inside is a source of security that the individual draws on to explore the broader environment with confidence (Counted, 2018; Devine-Wright et al., 2020). Significant places provide a smooth transition for people to explore both the inside (private) and outside (public) spaces. Public safety measures that were implemented in many countries to control the spread of SARS-CoV-2 have shifted the center point between the inside and outside of place. What is happening on the outside has somehow encroached the inside spaces of our homes where

---

[1] Ontological security is a psychological state derived from having a sense of continuity during a stressful life event (Gustafsson & Krickel-Choi, 2020).

privacy and safety are paramount. With many businesses and schools moving to online platforms, there has been a loss of privacy in the *inside* place. Working from home has made it challenging to protect inside spaces from aspects of life that usually occurred in outside spaces. Exploration of the outside space has been limited in many ways by community mitigation strategies that have restricted mobility (e.g., stay-at-home orders, physical distancing measures) and personal concerns about SARS-CoV-2 infection. These dialectical tensions disrupt the inside–outside balance and make it difficult for people to access places of attachment as havens of comfort and safety.

Fixity–Flow

Devine-Wright et al. (2020) proposed fixity–flow as a dialectic that explores the tension between the static and mobile aspects of our interactions with place. Fixity refers to the stable, anchored aspects of our subjective place experiences, whereas flow captures the unstable, mobile relations that people have with place. This perspective posits that our relationships with place are dynamically re-imagined as we navigate the public health crisis. In this dialectic, the fixities of place are interwoven with the dynamic flows of our shifting relationships with place. According to Devine-Wright et al. (2020), "mobilities re-signify fixities and vice versa" (p. 3). When we are fixed or confined to a particular place, it compels us to re-signify or re-value mobility (Di Masso et al., 2019). The COVID-19 pandemic has confined many people to their homes, a fixity that was largely prompted by stay-at-home orders and other social distancing regulations. Fixities are often followed by attempts to regain flow, such as when a person visits family living in another geographical location despite the lockdown laws that have been implemented.

Conversely, flow also re-signifies fixities. Widespread global transmission of SARS-CoV-2 has changed the way people choose their travel destinations. People may be less inclined to travel to destinations with a high burden of COVID-19, even though those locations may have been prominent tourist destinations before the public health crisis. People have become aware of the risks associated with traveling to specific destinations and are cautious about visiting COVID-19 hotspots that might be considered unsafe (The New York Times, 2021). This fixity–flow tension can create class-based and racialized patterns of place experiences (Devine-Wright et al., 2020). For example, socioeconomically disadvantaged communities have been stigmatized during the COVID-19 pandemic because of where they live (Jay et al., 2020). Thus, if we are to fully understand the effect of the public health crisis on place attachment, we must consider how constellations of fixity–flow shift the relationships that different people have with place.

Why Relationships with Place Matter in a Pandemic

The environmental psychology literature has long valued the relationships that people have with place. While drawing on the existing body of work on place attachment, recent perspectives have used the COVID-19 pandemic to expand our understanding of emplacement–displacement, inside–outside, and fixity–flow dialectics of place (Devine-Wright et al., 2020). Policymaking may also be informed by discourse that enriches the way that people-place bonds are appreciated and understood (Greenfield, 2012).

Different levels of policy may be influenced by exploring the changing nature of our relationships with place during the COVID-19 pandemic. Each of the place attachment domains (i.e., place, person, process) has direct policy implications. For example, information learned from the place dimension can be used to inform community-based policies centered on increasing accessibility to public spaces (e.g., parks, tourist sites) during and after a pandemic. The physical attributes of a place can help create access to long-term public amenities and infrastructure to improve the well-being of residents.

Information on how the pandemic has changed the person dimension is directly tied to policy at both local and national levels. For instance, post-pandemic funding could be allocated to boosting a city's cultural lifeforms after lockdown. Tourism incentives can be created to rekindle attachment bonds of people with cities and cultural sites. Policymakers can evaluate and monitor place attachment experiences of citizens to create or improve policies addressing social isolation and the health of affected communities. Broader policy implications may have to do with reconstructing place identity, especially for places that the COVID-19 pandemic has impacted immensely. For example, by March 2021, there were about one million COVID-19 cases and 30,564 deaths recorded in the city of New York alone (The New York Times, 2021). Although it is one of the most favored cities and destinations in the world, New York City may never be the same after the COVID-19 pandemic. The public health crisis has shifted the way New York City has been perceived in the media, with some news outlets referring to it as the *epicenter of the COVID-19 pandemic*. That stigma may be difficult to recover from, and it could also affect how people experience the city of New York in the future. Local policymakers may need to find innovative ways of rebranding the city and relaunching it to the world after the COVID-19 pandemic.

Policymakers must have the ability to capture the full impact of a pandemic on their cities and use that information to guide policy. Our work in this book concentrates on building a deeper understanding of how pandemics impact place attachment, human agency in accessing place, and the complexity of place experiences in the context of a pandemic. Our relationship with place and how it satiates our individual needs continue to evolve, especially during a global public health crisis (Weil, 2020). This book explores how the notion of people-place bonds has grown to include an understanding of what it means to live in a place that is undergoing rapid disruption (Counted et al., 2021; Weil, 2020).

Structure of the Book

This book rekindles the well-known connection between people and place in the context of a global pandemic. The chapters are divided into two sections. In the first section, *Place Attachment During a Pandemic*, we review the nature of the COVID-19 pandemic and the extent of its impact on place attachment and human–environment interactions. We examine how restrictions in mobility and environmental changes can have a significant psychological burden on people who are dealing with the effect of place attachment disruption that arises during a pandemic. This section starts with a scoping review in Chapter 2, which synthesizes empirical research that has focused on place attachment during the COVID-19 pandemic. Chapter 3 examines the relationship between place attachment and resource loss during a pandemic. The chapter addresses how resource loss during an experience of place attachment disruption can alter our experiences with places that are under the threat of a pandemic. In Chapter 4, we extend the notion of place attachment disruption as a distressing experience by exploring the potential for it to evoke a subjective state of distress that constitutes suffering. Chapter 5 uses John Bowlby's original thesis on attachment and loss to unpack the concept of place attachment disruption. We introduce and discuss a reparative model of place attachment disruption comprising three distinct but related phases—protest, despair, and detachment—that offer one way of understanding how disruption can be transformed into recovery.

In the second section, *Adjusting to Place Attachment Disruption During and After a Pandemic*, we focus on adaptive processes and responses that could enable people to adjust positively to place attachment disruption. Building on previous chapters that touch on resource loss and suffering, Chapter 6 describes how people can respond adaptively to resource loss that underlies a place attachment disruption by investing available resources and cultivating resilience despite what has been lost. Chapter 7 discusses the capacity for people to change place attachment disruption into a character-building process that facilitates both short-term adaptation and long-term well-being. We focus specifically on a trio of character strengths—gratitude, hope, and spirituality—that people could engage to strengthen and transcend their immediate experiences of attachment disruption and build psychospiritual capacities for dealing with future resource loss. In Chapter 8, we conclude the book by discussing the potential for pro-environmental behavior to promote place attachment and flourishing in the aftermath of the COVID-19 pandemic. We introduce an integrative framework of *place flourishing* and explore its post-pandemic implications for theory, research, policy, and practice.

This book draws on frameworks in environmental psychology, tourism, positive psychology, and health psychology. We consider the value of both old and new people-place relationships in contributing to a post-pandemic recovery plan by embodying experiences and practices of affective, cognitive, and behavioral significance. Based on lessons learned from the COVID-19 pandemic up to the time of writing, we share research and practical recommendations for post-pandemic recovery. Although many of the insights gleaned while writing this book have particularly strong relevance to the COVID-19 pandemic, we believe they could also prove useful to society as we prepare for and encounter future public health crises.

References

Ainsworth, M. S. (1989). Attachments beyond infancy. *American Psychologist, 44*(4), 709–716. https://doi.org/10.1037/0003-066X.44.4.709
Boğaç, C. (2009). Place attachment in a foreign settlement. *Journal of Environmental Psychology, 29*(2), 267–278. https://doi.org/10.1016/j.jenvp.2009.01.001
Bowlby, J. (1969). *Attachment and loss: Attachment* (Vol. 1). Basic Books.
Brown, B. B., & Perkins, D. D. (1992). Disruptions in place attachment. In I. Altman & S. M. Low (Eds.), *Place attachment* (pp. 279–304). Springer.
Captari, L. E., Hook, J. N., Aten, J. D., Davis, E. B., & Tisdale, T. C. (2019). Embodied spirituality following disaster: Exploring intersections of religious and place attachment in resilience and meaning-making. In V. Counted & F. Watts (Eds.), *The psychology of religion and place* (pp. 49–79). Palgrave Macmillan. https://doi.org/10.1007/978-3-030-28848-8_4
Cicirelli, V. G. (1991). Attachment theory in old age: Protection of the attached figure. In K. A. Pillemer & K. McCartney (Eds.), *Parent-child relations throughout life* (pp. 25–42). Lawrence Erlbaum Associates.
Cicirelli, V. G. (2004). God as the ultimate attachment figure for older adults. *Attachment & Human Development, 6*(4), 371–388. https://doi.org/10.1080/1461673042000303091
Counted, V. (2016). Making sense of place attachment: Towards a holistic understanding of people-place relationships and experiences. *Environment, Space, Place, 8*(1), 7–32. https://doi.org/10.5840/esplace2016811
Counted, V. (2018). The Circle of Place Spirituality (CoPS): Towards an attachment and exploration motivational systems approach in the psychology of religion. In A. Village & R. W. Hood (Eds.), *Research in the social scientific study of religion* (Vol. 29, pp. 145–174). Brill. https://doi.org/10.1163/9789004382640_009
Counted, V., & Zock, H. T. (2019). Place spirituality: An attachment perspective. *Archive for the Psychology of Religion, 41*(1), 12–25. https://doi.org/10.1177/0084672419833448
Counted, V., Neff, M. A., Captari, L. E., & Cowden, R. G. (2021). Transcending place attachment disruptions during a public health crisis: Spiritual struggles, resilience, and transformation. *Journal of Psychology and Christianity, 39*(4), 276–286.
Counted, V., Pargament, K. I., Bechara, A. O., Joynt, S., & Cowden, R. G. (2020). Hope and well-being in vulnerable contexts during the COVID-19 pandemic: Does religious coping matter? *The Journal of Positive Psychology*. Advance online publication. https://doi.org/10.1080/17439760.2020.1832247
Cowden, R. G., Davis, E. B., Counted, V., Chen, Y., Rueger, S. Y., VanderWeele, T. J., Lemke, A. W., Glowiak, K. J., & Worthington, E. L., Jr. (2021). Suffering, mental health, and psychological well-being during the COVID-19 pandemic: A longitudinal study of U.S. adults with chronic health conditions. *Wellbeing, Space and Society, 2*, 100048. https://doi.org/10.1016/j.wss.2021.100048
Devine-Wright, P., de Carvalho, L. P., Di Masso, A., Lewicka, M., Manzo, L., & Williams, D. R. (2020). "Re-placed"—Reconsidering relationships with place and lessons from a pandemic. *Journal of Environmental Psychology, 72*, 101514. https://doi.org/10.1016/j.jenvp.2020.101514
Di Masso, A., Williams, D. R., Raymond, C. M., Buchecker, M., Degenhardt, B., Devine-Wright, P., Hertzog, A., Lewicka, M., Manzo, L., Shahrad, A., Stedman, R., Verbrugge, L., & von Wirth, T. (2019). Between fixities and flows: Navigating place attachments in an increasingly

mobile world. *Journal of Environmental Psychology, 61*, 125–133. https://doi.org/10.1016/j.jenvp.2019.01.006

Fornara, F., Bonaiuto, M., & Bonnes, M. (2010). Cross-validation of abbreviated perceived residential environment quality (PREQ) and neighborhood attachment (NA) indicators. *Environment and Behavior, 42*(2), 171–196. https://doi.org/10.1177/0013916508330998

Giuliani, M. V. (2003). Theory of attachment and place attachment. In M. Bonnes, T. Lee, & M. Bonaiuto (Eds.), *Psychological theories for environmental issues* (pp. 137–170). Ashgate.

Govender, K., Cowden, R. G., Nyamaruze, P., Armstrong, R. M., & Hatane, L. (2020). Beyond the disease: Contextualized implications of the COVID-19 pandemic for children and young people living in Eastern and Southern Africa. *Frontiers in Public Health, 8*, 504. https://doi.org/10.3389/fpubh.2020.00504

Granqvist, P. (2020). *Attachment in religion and spirituality: A wider view*. Guilford Press.

Greenfield, E. A. (2012). Using ecological frameworks to advance a field of research, practice, and policy on aging-in-place initiatives. *The Gerontologist, 52*(1), 1–12. https://doi.org/10.1093/geront/gnr108

Gustafsson, K., & Krickel-Choi, N. C. (2020). Returning to the roots of ontological security: Insights from the existentialist anxiety literature. *European Journal of International Relations, 26*(3), 875–895. https://doi.org/10.1177/1354066120927073

Heidegger, M. (1958). An ontological consideration of place (J. T. Wilde & W. Kluback, Trans.). In M. Heidegger (Ed.), *The question of being* (pp. 18–27). Twayne Publishers.

Honey-Rosés, J., Anguelovski, I., Chireh, V. K., Daher, C., Konijnendijk van den Bosch, C., Litt, J. S., Mawani, V., McCall, M. K., Orellana, A., Oscilowicz, E., Sánchez, U., Senbel, M., Tan, X., Villagomez, E., Zapata, O., & Nieuwenhuijsen, M. J. (2020). The impact of COVID-19 on public space: An early review of the emerging questions—Design, perceptions and inequities. *Cities & Health*. Advance online publication. https://doi.org/10.1080/23748834.2020.1780074

Jay, J., Bor, J., Nsoesie, E. O., Lipson, S. K., Jones, D. K., Galea, S., & Raifman, J. (2020). Neighbourhood income and physical distancing during the COVID-19 pandemic in the United States. *Nature Human Behaviour, 4*(12), 1294–1302. https://doi.org/10.1038/s41562-020-00998-2

Jorgensen, B. S., & Stedman, R. C. (2001). Sense of place as an attitude: Lakeshore owners attitudes toward their properties. *Journal of Environmental Psychology, 21*(3), 233–248. https://doi.org/10.1006/jevp.2001.0226

Kunstler, J. H. (1993). *The geography of nowhere. The rise and decline of America's man-made landscape*. Touchstone.

Lewicka, M. (2008). Place attachment, place identity, and place memory: Restoring the forgotten city past. *Journal of Environmental Psychology, 28*(3), 209–231. https://doi.org/10.1016/j.jenvp.2008.02.001

Lewicka, M. (2010). What makes a neighborhood different from home and city? Effects of place scale on place attachment. *Journal of Environmental Psychology, 30*(1), 35–51. https://doi.org/10.1016/j.jenvp.2009.05.004

Lewicka, M. (2011). Place attachment: How far have we come in the last 40 years? *Journal of Environmental Psychology, 31*(3), 207–230. https://doi.org/10.1016/j.jenvp.2010.10.001

Low, S. M., & Altman, I. (1992). Place attachment: A conceptual inquiry. In I. Altman & S. M. Low (Eds.), *Place attachment* (pp. 1–12). Springer. https://doi.org/10.1007/978-1-4684-8753-4_1

Manzo, L. C. (2003). Beyond house and haven: Toward a revisioning of emotional relationship with places. *Journal of Environmental Psychology, 23*(1), 47–61. https://doi.org/10.1016/S0272-4944(02)00074-9

Marcheschi, E., Laike, T., Brunt, D., Hansson, L., & Johansson, M. (2015). Quality of life and place attachment among people with severe mental illness. *Journal of Environmental Psychology, 41*, 145–154. https://doi.org/10.1016/j.jenvp.2014.12.003

Ng, C. F. (1998). Canada as a new place: The immigrant's experience. *Journal of Environmental Psychology, 18*(1), 55–67. https://doi.org/10.1006/jevp.1997.0065

Proshansky, H. M., Fabian, A. K., & Kaminoff, R. (1983). Place-identity: Physical world socialization of the self. *Journal of Environmental Psychology, 3*(1), 57–83. https://doi.org/10.1016/S0272-4944(83)80021-8

Raymond, C. M., Brown, G., & Weber, D. (2010). The measurement of place attachment: Personal, community, and environmental connections. *Journal of Environmental Psychology, 30*(4), 422–434. https://doi.org/10.1016/j.jenvp.2010.08.002

Relph, E. (1976). *Place and placelessness* (Vol. 67). Pion.

Rollero, C., & De Piccoli, N. (2010). Place attachment, identification and environment perception: An empirical study. *Journal of Environmental Psychology, 30*(2), 198–205. https://doi.org/10.1016/j.jenvp.2009.12.003

Scannell, L., & Gifford, R. (2010). Defining place attachment: A tripartite organizing framework. *Journal of Environmental Psychology, 30*(1), 1–10. https://doi.org/10.1016/j.jenvp.2009.09.006

Scannell, L., & Gifford, R. (2014). Comparing the theories of interpersonal and place attachment. In L. C. Manzo & P. Devine-Wright (Eds.), *Place attachment: Advances in theory, methods, and applications* (pp. 23–36). Routledge.

Scannell, L., & Gifford, R. (2017). Place attachment enhances psychological need satisfaction. *Environment and Behavior, 49*(4), 359–389. https://doi.org/10.1177/0013916516637648

Seamon, D. (2012). Place, place identity, and phenomenology: A triadic interpretation based on JG Bennett's systematics. In H. Casakin & F. Bernardo (Eds.), *The role of place identity in the perception, understanding, and design of built environments* (pp. 3–21). Bentham Books.

Sheldrake, R. (2019). Sacred places: The presence of the past. In V. Counted & F. Watts (Eds.), *The psychology of religion and place* (pp. 15–31). Palgrave Macmillan. https://doi.org/10.1007/978-3-030-28848-8_2

The New York Times. (2021, March 24). New York coronavirus map and case count. *The New York Times*. Retrieved from https://www.nytimes.com/interactive/2020/us/new-york-coronavirus-cases.html

Turner, B. S. (2010). Enclosures, enclaves, and entrapment. *Sociological Inquiry, 80*(2), 241–260. https://doi.org/10.1111/j.1475-682X.2010.00329.x

Weil, J. (2020). Pandemic place: Assessing domains of the person-place fit measure for older adults (PPFM-OA) during COVID-19. *Journal of Aging & Social Policy*. Advance online publication. https://doi.org/10.1080/08959420.2020.1824539

Part I
Place Attachment During a Pandemic

Chapter 2
Place Attachment During the COVID-19 Pandemic: A Scoping Review

Victor Counted, Richard G. Cowden, and Haywantee Ramkissoon

Contents

Method... 16
   Research Question... 16
   Inclusion Criteria... 16
   Literature Search... 17
   Screening and Selection.. 17
   Data Extraction and Synthesis.. 19
Results and Discussion.. 19
   Study Characteristics... 19
   Summary of Findings.. 20
Implications for Research and Practice... 28
Strengths and Limitations.. 30
Conclusion... 31
References... 31

Early reports in 2021 show that the COVID-19 pandemic has affected many people, communities, and societies (Huang et al., 2021). Interactions and bonds with places that are a valued part of our lives have also been impacted by the public health crisis (Counted et al., 2021; Devine-Wright et al., 2020). People have been emplaced in their homes and displaced from places of significance, in part because of stay-at-home orders that were implemented to control the spread of SARS-CoV-2 (Devine-Wright et al., 2020).

    Emplacement and displacement experiences during the COVID-19 pandemic have contributed to changes in the emotional connections that people have with their environments (Devine-Wright et al., 2020; Meagher & Cheadle, 2020; Stieger et al., 2021). Ramkissoon (2020) used the term *place confinement* to describe the way that people have been confined to their homes in order to control or limit transmission of SARS-CoV-2. Place confinement within the context of the COVID-19 pandemic has restricted people from accessing, interacting, and connecting with the broader environment, which can have consequences for mental, physical, spiritual, and social well-being (Counted et al., 2021; Meagher & Cheadle, 2020; Ramkissoon, 2020). However, some empirical research suggests that place confinement may be a generative experience because it can foster or reinforce attachment to one's home. For example, social (e.g., kinship, family members) and physical (e.g., interior design, restorations) features of people's homes have been among the predictors of place attachment during the COVID-19 pandemic (Meagher & Cheadle, 2020).

Although research addressing the impact of the public health crisis on human–environment interactions is ongoing, taking stock of the existing evidence on people-place relationships during the COVID-19 pandemic could help to inform future research and relevant policies. Based on a preliminary search performed in PubMed, PROSPERO, PsycINFO, and Web of Science databases during September 2020, we did not identify any scoping or systematic reviews focusing on people-place relationships during the COVID-19 pandemic. In this chapter, we perform a scoping review to synthesize and descriptively map empirical research on place attachment within the context of the COVID-19 pandemic. We discuss the implications of the findings for research and policymaking decisions centered on promoting post-pandemic recovery.

Method

This review was conducted in accordance with the Joanna Briggs Institute (JBI) methodology for scoping reviews (Peters et al., 2020).

Research Question

We formalized a research question that was developed by integrating themes from preliminary searches and our own expertise about people-place relationships. Based on this process, the overarching research question of interest in this scoping review is what empirical evidence has been documented on place attachment within the context of the COVID-19 pandemic?

Inclusion Criteria

Participants Clinical and nonclinical samples comprising individuals of any age, gender, and race/ethnicity who lived through the COVID-19 pandemic that emerged in late 2019.

Concept The phenomenon of interest was place attachment, which is a term that is used to describe the emotional bonds that people have with places in the environment (Scannell & Gifford, 2017). Given that scholars sometimes define and operationalize place attachment differently, we included all studies that explicitly addressed or measured place attachment.

Context Studies conducted in any geographic location and setting that were impacted by the COVID-19 pandemic.

Types of Sources We included qualitative, quantitative, and mixed-methods studies published in peer-reviewed journals. Dissertations, conference or meeting abstracts, case studies, commentaries, reviews, and other scholarly articles and book chapters with no reported data were excluded. Eligible publications were restricted to those in the English language.

Literature Search

The literature search followed a three-step search process outlined in the JBI Manual for Evidence Synthesis (Peters et al., 2020). We initially generated a list of potential search terms by screening the titles, abstracts, and index terms of peer-reviewed published papers that were identified following a limited search that was performed in the PsycINFO and PubMed databases. Using those search terms, we undertook a series of secondary electronic searches in Embase, PsycARTICLES, PsycINFO, PubMed, and Web of Science databases to identify relevant published articles. The final database searches were performed on 31 March 2021, which included all available records from 1 January 2020 up to the search date. The search strategy that we used in the PubMed database is detailed in Table 2.1. The format of search expressions was modified to fit the search specifications of the different database interfaces.

Screening and Selection

In the second step of the search process, we imported the published peer-reviewed studies that were retrieved during the database search procedure into Covidence and removed duplicate records. The first author screened the titles and abstracts of all records for eligibility. The second author independently completed the same title and abstract screening process with a random sample of 25% of the records. Both reviewers retrieved and screened the remaining full-text records against the eligibility criteria. They also performed the final step of ensuring that literature saturation was achieved by searching the reference lists of eligible studies to determine whether any previously unidentified articles met the criteria for inclusion in the review. Disagreements between the two reviewers at each stage were resolved via consensus.

Table 2.1 Electronic databases, search terms, and sample search strategy

Databases	Search terms		Search strategy (PubMed)
	Group A	Group B	
Embase	Coronavirus	Place attachment	#1: ("coronavirus" [title/abstract] OR "corona virus" [title/abstract] OR "covid-19" [title/abstract] OR "covid19" [title/abstract] OR "2019-ncov" [title/abstract] OR "sars-cov-2" [title/abstract])
PsycARTICLES	Corona virus	Home attachment	
PsycINFO	Covid-19	Sense of place	
PubMed	Covid19	Place identity	
Web of Science	2019-ncov	Place affect	#2: ("place attachment" [title/abstract] OR "home attachment" [title/abstract] OR "sense of place" [title/abstract] OR "place identity" [title/abstract] OR "place affect" [title/abstract] OR "place dependence" [title/abstract] OR "people-place relation*" [title/abstract] OR "place attachment disruption" [title/abstract] OR "place disruption" [title/abstract] OR "displacement" [title/abstract] OR "emplacement" [title/abstract] OR "place confinement" [title/abstract] OR "home confinement" [title/abstract] OR "homebound" [title/abstract])
	Sars-cov-2	Place dependence	
		Home attachment	
		People-place relation*	
		Place attachment disruption	
		Place disruption	
		Displacement	
		Emplacement	
		Place confinement	
		Home confinement homebound	#3: #1 AND #2

Note. Embase Excerpta Medica Database, *PsycINFO* Psychology Information

Data Extraction and Synthesis

The data extraction procedure was consistent with best practice guidelines (see Peters et al., 2020; Tricco et al., 2018). The first two authors independently extracted and entered relevant data into an Excel spreadsheet for storage and management. The information that was extracted included publication details (i.e., lead author, year), context (i.e., country of origin, study purpose[s], study population[s]), research methodology (i.e., design, date[s] of data collection, sample size, age and sex of participants), and the primary results(s). The extracted data from both reviewers were cross-checked and inconsistencies were resolved through consultation with one another. The extracted data from each of the included studies were tabulated.

Results and Discussion

A visual display of the study screening and selection process is presented in a Preferred Reporting Items for Systematic Reviews and Meta-Analyses extension for Scoping Reviews (PRISMA-ScR) flow diagram (see Fig. 2.1). After removing duplicates, the electronic database searches yielded a total of 394 unique records that were potentially relevant. The record screening and assessment procedure revealed that 388 records did not meet the eligibility criteria. There were six published articles that met the criteria for inclusion in the review, all of which are included in the references (Cohen et al., 2020; Kala, 2021; Kamata, 2021; Meagher & Cheadle, 2020; Tilaki et al., 2021; Wang et al., 2020). The extracted data from each of the included studies are reported in Table 2.2.

Study Characteristics

An equal number of studies were published in 2020 and 2021. Most of the studies were conducted in countries within Asia, including one each in China, India, Israel, Japan, and Malaysia. The other study was conducted in the US. The studies each employed a quantitative research design, all of which were observational. Five studies were cross-sectional, and one study used a longitudinal design. All studies included samples from nonclinical populations. When researchers targeted specific subpopulations, they focused on residents or vendors living within geographic locations that were of interest. Study samples were almost exclusively adults. Children were not represented in any of the studies, but a small proportion of adolescents were included in one study. Sample sizes ranged from 144 to 1458. Both gender groups were represented in each study.

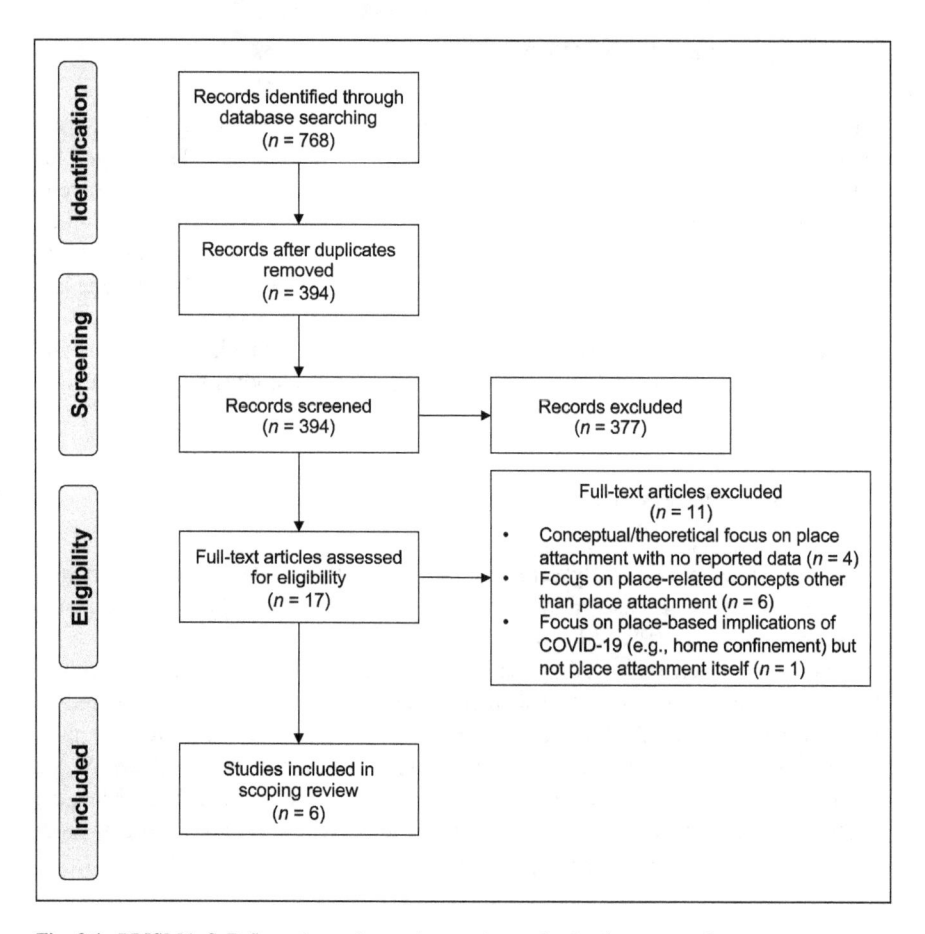

Fig. 2.1 PRISMA-ScR flow chart of record screening and selection protocol

Summary of Findings

We evaluated the scope of the included studies and summarized the findings under two common themes that are relevant to the research question on place attachment within the context of the COVID-19 pandemic, namely (1) place attachment and well-being and (2) place attachment and tourism.

Place Attachment and Well-being In the single longitudinal study we identified, Meagher and Cheadle (2020) examined the mental health implications of home attachment during the early phase of the COVID-19 pandemic in a sample of US adults. Using three waves of data with measurements taken 2 weeks apart from one another, the authors found that kinship (e.g., togetherness), stimulation (e.g., entertainment), and restorative ambiances (e.g., tranquility) of people's homes were associated with higher levels of home attachment during the COVID-19 pandemic. Home attachment at Wave 1 was associated with lower levels of subsequent depression, anxiety, and stress at Wave 2, suggesting that a person's bond with their home

Table 2.2 Summary of extracted characteristics for all included studies ($n = 6$)

Publication details		Context			Research methodology						Primary result(s) and key findings
Lead author	Year	Country of origin	Study purpose(s)	Study population(s)	Design	Date(s) of data collection	Sample size	Sex	Age		
Cohen	2020	Israel	Examine the role of healthcare services in promoting community resilience of urban and suburban communities during the COVID-19 pandemic	Adult residents of two Arab communities in Israel	Quantitative (cross-sectional)	May 2020	196 (UC = 112) (SC = 84)	67.9% ♀ (UC) 67.9% ♀ (SC)	$M = 31.5 \pm 15.1$ (UC) $M = 39.7 \pm 11.9$ (SC)		• After statistically controlling for sociodemographic factors, community resilience in the SC ($M = 3.37$) was significantly higher ($p < .05$) than in the UC ($M = 3.08$) – When specific community resilience factors were examined, group differences were primarily due to higher levels of preparedness and place attachment in the SC **Key finding:** Community preparedness and place attachment were the major components that distinguished the perceived resilience of urban and suburban communities during the COVID-19 pandemic

Table 2.2 (continued)

Publication details		Context		Research methodology					Primary result(s) and key findings
Lead author	Year	Country of origin	Study purpose(s)	Study population(s)	Design	Date(s) of data collection	Sample size	Sex	Age	
Meagher	2020	US	Examine (1) associations of home ambiances (i.e., restoration, kinship, stimulation) with home attachment, and (2) associations of home attachment with changes in depression, anxiety, and perceived stress during the initial wave of the COVID-19 pandemic	General adult population of the US (recruited via MTurk)	Quantitative (longitudinal, 3 waves each separated by 2 weeks)	March and April 2020	289 (baseline)	46% ♀	$M = 37.4 \pm 11.6$	• After statistically controlling for sociodemographic factors and personality traits, multilevel modeling indicated that the ambiances of kinship ($\beta = .11$), stimulation ($\beta = .13$), and restoration ($\beta = .26$) each associated positively with home attachment (all p-values < .01) – Association between kinship ambience and home attachment increased over time ($\beta = .06, p < .05$) • Cross-lagged panel analyses revealed that Wave 1 home attachment was associated with lower depression ($\beta = -.10$), anxiety ($\beta = -.11$), and stress ($\beta = -.09$) at Wave 2 (all p-values < .05) – Associations of home attachment at Wave 2 with all three mental health outcomes at Wave 3 were negligible (all p-values > .05) – Perceived stress at Wave 2 was associated with lower levels of home attachment at Wave 3 ($\beta = -.09, p < .05$) **Key finding:** Home attachment was particularly important during the initial phase of the US national response to the SARS-CoV-2 outbreak

Publication details		Context		Research methodology					Primary result(s) and key findings
Lead author	Year	Country of origin	Study purpose(s)	Study population(s)	Design	Date(s) of data collection	Sample size	Sex	Age	
Wang	2020	China	Explore tourism risk perception as a mechanism linking place image depicted in anti-epidemic music videos, place attachment, and travel intention during the COVID-19 pandemic	General population of adolescents and adults who were not residents of Wuhan, China	Quantitative (cross-sectional)	March 2020	945	52.4% ♀	< 18 years (4.7%) 18–25 years (26%) 26–30 years (32.7%) 31–40 years (23.6%) 41–50 years (11.1%) 51–60 years (1.7%)	• After statistically controlling for sociodemographic factors: – Place image depicted in anti-epidemic music videos associated negatively with tourism risk perception ($\beta = -.36, p < .001$) – Tourism risk perception associated negatively with place attachment ($\beta = -.48, p < .001$) and travel intention ($\beta = -.57, p < .001$) – Place attachment associated positively with travel intention ($\beta = -.85, p < .001$) • Tourism risk perception partially mediated the associations of place images depicted in anti-epidemic music videos with both place attachment and travel intention • Associations of tourism risk perception with place attachment and travel intention were stronger among participants who had visited Wuhan in the past **Key finding:** Exposure to positive images about a travel destination in the media could lower a person's perceived risk of traveling to the location during a public health crisis, which may subsequently increase place attachment and travel intentions

(continued)

Table 2.2 (continued)

Publication details		Context			Research methodology					Primary result(s) and key findings
Lead author	Year	Country of origin	Study purpose(s)	Study population(s)	Design	Date(s) of data collection	Sample size	Sex	Age	
Kala	2021	India	Examine associations of religious motivation, spiritual beliefs, place attachment, and destination image with intentions to visit religious destinations after the COVID-19 pandemic	General adult population of India	Quantitative (cross-sectional)	September and October 2020	237	41.1% ♀	< 20 years (13.1%) 21–30 years (42.2%) 31–40 years (28.7%) 41–50 years (6.7%) > 50 years (9.3%)	• Structural equation modeling results indicated that religious motivation ($\beta = .51$), spiritual beliefs ($\beta = .61$), place attachment ($\beta = .52$), and destination image ($\beta = .67$) were each associated with greater intention to visit a religious destination (all p-values < .001) **Key finding:** Place attachment may be an important factor that influences whether a person is willing to visit a religious destination after the COVID-19 pandemic

Publication details		Context		Research methodology					Primary result(s) and key findings
Lead author	Year	Country of origin	Study purpose(s)	Study population(s)	Design	Date(s) of data collection	Sample size	Sex	Age	
Kamata	2021	Japan	Examine local residents' attitudes toward tourism during and after the COVID-19 pandemic	Adult residents of four well-known tourist destinations in Japan	Quantitative (cross-sectional)	September 2020	1458	48.8% ♀	20–29 years (3.6%) 30–39 years (11.9%) 40–49 years (28.1%) 50–59 years (31.4%) 60–69 years (18.6%) > 69 years (6.4%)	• Results from a structural equation model for acceptance of tourists during the COVID-19 pandemic indicated that: – Place attachment and perceived distinctiveness of place each associated positively with perceived positive impact of tourism in the regions (β = .27 to .28, both p-values < .001), which in turn was associated with more supportive attitudes toward future tourism development (β = .31, p < .001) – Place attachment associated negatively with perceived negative impact of tourism in the regions (β = –.13, p < .001), whereas the association for perceived distinctiveness was positive (β = .49, p < .001). In turn, perceived negative impact of tourism was associated with less supportive attitudes toward future tourism development (β = –.18, p < .001) – Place attachment associated positively with supportive attitudes toward future tourism development (β = .33, p < .001), but perceived distinctiveness of place did not (β = .03, p > .05) • A similar pattern of findings emerged when the structural equation model addressed acceptance of tourists after the COVID-19 pandemic **Key finding:** Perceptions and experiences of place (particularly place attachment) among local residents may affect their attitudes toward tourism and its impact both during and after the COVID-19 pandemic

Table 2.2 (continued)

Publication details		Context			Research methodology					Primary result(s) and key findings
Lead author	Year	Country of origin	Study purpose(s)	Study population(s)	Design	Date(s) of data collection	Sample size	Sex	Age	
Tilaki	2021	Malaysia	Examine night market vendors' attitudes and perceptions of tourism during the COVID-19 pandemic	Adult vendors operating at night markets in Penang, Malaysia	Quantitative (cross-sectional)	September 2020	144	43.1% ♀	$M = 45.0 \pm 14.5$	• After statistically adjusting for economic gain through tourism and community involvement, structural equation modeling results revealed that: – Place attachment associated positively with positive perceptions about tourism ($\beta = .24$, $p < .001$), but its association with negative perceptions about tourism was negligible ($\beta = .08$, $p > .05$) – The association between place attachment and tourism receptiveness was fully mediated by positive perceptions about tourism **Key finding:** Vendors' attachment to the night markets where they operate may have implications for their perceptions of tourists during the COVID-19 pandemic and openness to having tourists return to the destination once the public health crisis wanes

Note. COVID-19 coronavirus disease 2019, *M* mean, *MTurk* Amazon's Mechanical Turk, *SARS-CoV-2* severe acute respiratory syndrome coronavirus 2, *SC* suburban community, *UC* urban community, ♀ female may buffer against the effects of a global pandemic on psychological distress. These findings indicate that even though the public health crisis has disrupted connections with outdoor environments, many people may have derived benefits from rekindling or strengthening bonds with their homes. This narrative echoes the inside–outside dialectic that has been emphasized during the COVID-19 pandemic (Devine-Wright et al., 2020), which asserts that while the public health crisis has redefined our connection to the outside place it has also created opportunities for *inside* place experiences within our homes and places of refuge (Devine-Wright et al., 2020; see also Chapter 1).

Looking beyond the implications of the COVID-19 pandemic for individuals, one cross-sectional study compared the community resilience resources of suburban and urban communities in Israel (Cohen et al., 2020). Participants in the suburban community reported higher levels of overall community resilience resources compared to those in the urban community. The difference between the two samples was largely due to the perceived preparedness of community healthcare services during the public health crisis and strength of place attachment (Cohen et al., 2020). These findings highlight the need for residents of urban communities to build a sense of attachment to the places they live, which could be an important resilience resource that sustains well-being during a pandemic. There may be value in addressing issues of place inequality and fostering place attachment as a resource that could support positive adjustment amid public health crises.

Place Attachment and Tourism Two cross-sectional studies examined associations between place attachment and travel intentions during the COVID-19 pandemic. Kala (2021) explored whether place attachment among citizens of India might influence their willingness to visit religious destinations both during and after the public health crisis. The results indicated that people with higher levels of place attachment were more willing to visit religious destinations. In addition to place attachment itself, religious motivation and spiritual beliefs (including those pertaining to religious places) were both positively associated with intentions to visit religious places. These findings resonate with place spirituality theory, which emphasizes the many ways that religious/spiritual experiences are embedded in or facilitated by the relationships that people have with places (Counted, 2018; Counted & Zock, 2019). Even though there may be risks associated with traveling to religious destinations during the COVID-19 pandemic, it is possible that participants were motivated to visit religious places because physical closeness to a sacred geographical object of attachment may bring about a sense of security during a global pandemic (Billig, 2019).

Wang et al. (2020) examined the association between digital place images of a potential travel destination and risk perceptions among Chinese participants during the COVID-19 pandemic. The results revealed that place attachment associated positively with travel intention but negatively with tourism risk perceptions. The perceived risk of traveling to the city of Wuhan, China mediated the association between media place images depicted in anti-pandemic music videos and place attachment. These findings suggest that using technology to view positive images of a place that has been impacted by the public health crisis may lower the perceived risk of traveling to that location, which could lead to an increase in the person's sense of connection to that place. One takeaway from Wang et al.'s (2020) study is that place-related imagery could be a fruitful avenue for building more positive perceptions of cities that have experienced a high burden of COVID-19. Using digital media to disseminate positive images about cities and destinations around the world could boost tourism again and contribute to post-pandemic recovery.

Two studies explored place attachment and tourism receptiveness within the context of the COVID-19 pandemic. Kamata (2021) examined local Japanese residents' attitudes toward tourism both during and after the public health crisis. The findings indicated that place attachment associated positively with perceived positive impact of tourism and supportive attitudes toward future tourism. Hence, the way that residents view and experience their environment can affect their attitudes toward tourism. Similarly, Tilaki et al. (2021) investigated the association between Malaysian night market vendors' place attitudes and their perceptions of tourism during the public health crisis. They found that the relation between place attachment and tourism receptiveness was fully mediated by positive perceptions about tourism. Informal vendors are a part of the fascination that visitors have about a geographical place because they showcase regional culture and often play a role in the local experiences of tourists. Identifying ways to support informal local vendors might help relaunch tourism after the COVID-19 pandemic.

Implications for Research and Practice

The studies included in this scoping review offer insight into place attachment experiences within the context of the COVID-19 pandemic. Our findings suggest that scholars have principally dedicated empirical efforts toward links between place attachment, well-being, and tourism. We reflect on the broader implications of these findings for research and practice addressing people-place relationships.

In a world where the tourism industry has been impacted by a global pandemic, people may be able to maintain some sense of connection to places of attachment through virtual tools and technologies (e.g., positive media images of significant places). Virtual tools make it possible to "visit" places in a way that may contribute to sustaining place relations when access to the physical place is limited (Devine-Wright et al., 2020). Media promotion could be used as a mechanism to rebuild the tourism industry by digitally reminding people of places that are significant to them and possibly reduce their sense of alienation from destinations they value. Media images could encourage people to travel and help re-establish attachment to places again (Wang et al., 2020). Digital images that highlight the safety protocols which are being implemented at religious destinations could reduce the distress associated with traveling to those places, as people may feel compelled by their religious traditions to travel to sacred places despite the risk of SARS-CoV-2 infection. Hence, religious institutions and destinations need to be given the kind of support that enables them to provide opportunities for people to safely access sacred spaces.

Based on the findings of this review, governments and policy makers ought to adopt policies that recognize place as a mechanism that can contribute to resource building and may facilitate resilience in times of disaster. This may include budgeting for initiatives that bring communities together in places to share experiences and bond with one another before disaster hits, which could assist people with cultivating community-based resources that enable them to more effectively respond to and recover from disaster. For example, supporting religious communities, community events, and activities that bring people together in a place can go a long way toward strengthening people's place bonds. This notion must not be limited to the COVID-19 pandemic but should be applied to disasters in general. The current public health crisis has taught us that people-place relationships must be part of the public health discourse. If the highest levels of human flourishing are to be achieved before, during, and after any major disaster that affects society's capacity to interact with the broader environment, the implications of people-place relationships for individual and community well-being ought to be addressed in public health policies and decision-making (see Chapter 8).

The COVID-19 pandemic has also disrupted community-level aspects of life (e.g., healthcare services, faith community, community connectedness, community services) that often intersect the relationships we have with places (Bentley et al., 2020; Cohen et al., 2020; Fenton et al., 2020). The impact of future disasters on communities could be reduced by equipping them with resources that strengthen their collective sense of place attachment (Cohen et al., 2020). Some evidence from the COVID-19 pandemic suggests that creating spaces for community interactions and activities can strengthen people's sense of community and place attachment. In one study, Fenton et al. (2020) found that interactions within online sport communities helped fans to sustain their sense of connection to the cities where their favorite sports teams were located. Community-level aspects of life can play an important role in strengthening people's relationships with place, and activities that focus on community interactions can be harnessed to foster stronger place attachment.

Digital technologies may be useful tools for facilitating experiential therapies that enable people to adapt to their physical place attachment disruptions (Counted et al., 2021; Thompson-de Benoit & Kramer, 2020). Specific kinds of digital technologies (e.g., virtual reality) could allow people to virtually experience physical places that are valued and meaningful to them, even though access to the physical environment may be limited. Virtual experiences of places allow a person to transcend the "physical thresholds of confinement, thereby breaking the spatial and social boundaries imposed by fixity, and mitigating negative feelings of displacement associated with confinement at home" (Devine-Wright et al., 2020, p. 5). Although the virtual experience of a place may be the temporary geography of its physical reality, the use of virtual spaces for leisure may decrease as people begin to look for online shopping experiences and platforms to have formal meetings (Paköz et al., 2021). Through the creation of virtual spaces where people can bridge the divide between place and mobility, spatially fixed aspects of our place experiences have been replaced by fluidity in people-place relationships. As we come to realize that the outside space is no longer available as it formerly was, the inside space may be re-signified as a place where people use virtual means to escape and engage in everyday activities. Future studies exploring the various roles of technology in facilitating community interactions, mobility, and resilience can help expand our understanding of how technology could be used to support people-place relationships during an environmental disaster.

Public health crises teach us that in the face of imminent danger we can abruptly change our behavior by adjusting to the social expectations of our environments (Counted et al., 2021). Scientists around the world have acquired a wealth of knowledge about the challenges of conducting research amid a global disaster. It is important that scholars take the lessons that have been learned to prepare for and improve upon research involving disasters, particularly research on place-related concepts that are often affected by natural and man-made disasters (e.g., place attachment).

Strengths and Limitations

This scoping review used best practice guidelines to systematically identify and synthesize research on place attachment during the COVID-19 pandemic. Although the findings are an important step in refining our understanding of how the public health crisis has affected people-place relationships, we acknowledge two key limitations of this review. First, the focus of this scoping review was exclusively on place attachment. People-place concepts tend to vary across disciplines, and the place attachment construct appears more prominently in the social science literature. Moreover, the COVID-19 pandemic has impacted many dimensions of place that extend beyond place attachment. For example, we identified several studies that focused on other concepts (e.g., place confinement) that provide insight into how the public health crisis has affected well-being. Given the scope of this book and our emphasis on the bonds that people have with places, those kinds of studies did not form part of this review. Nonetheless, this scoping review offers a useful summary of existing research on place attachment during the public health crisis and serves as a foundation for subsequent reviews on other important place-related concepts. Second, we did not include an assessment of study quality in this scoping review. Scoping reviews are not usually accompanied by an evaluation of the quality of evidence evaluation (Khalil et al., 2016), but concerns have been raised about the quality of scientific outputs during the COVID-19 pandemic because of how much research has been conducted and published on the topic in such a short period of time (Guinart & de Filippis, 2020; Parmar, 2020). To illustrate, most of the studies included in this review were cross-sectional. Thus, our understanding of the cause-and-effect associations between place attachment and the variables that formed part of the studies that were reviewed is severely limited. Our knowledge about place attachment within the context of the COVID-19 pandemic and other disasters could be greatly enhanced through research that employs methodologically rigorous designs and analytic approaches.

Conclusion

The COVID-19 pandemic has laid bare the disruptive nature of global health crises. Society has been forced to consider and redefine the emplacement–displacement, fixity–flow, and inside–outside dynamics that have usually been applied to people-place relationships. To gain insight into the way that the current public health crisis has affected people relationships, this scoping review synthesized empirical evidence that has been reported on place attachment during the COVID-19 pandemic. The findings revealed that place attachment may support well-being in times of disaster and could be used to promote tourism in the aftermath of chronic global public health crises. Although further research is needed to build on the place attachment research that has been published so far on the COVID-19 pandemic, the findings of this scoping review can be used to inform future research and practice addressing people-place relationships during the current health pandemic and other disasters that emerge in the future.

References

Bentley, J. A., Mohamed, F., Feeny, N., Ahmed, L. B., Musa, K., Tubeec, A. M., Angula, D., Egeh, M. H., & Zoellner, L. (2020). Local to global: Somali perspectives on faith, community, and resilience in response to COVID-19. *Psychological Trauma: Theory, Research, Practice, and Policy, 12*(S1), S261–S263. https://doi.org/10.1037/tra0000854

Billig, M. (2019). 'To him I commit my spirit': Attachment to god, the land and the people as a means of dealing with crises in Gaza Strip. In V. Counted & F. Watts (Eds.), *The psychology of religion and place* (pp. 219–238). Palgrave Macmillan. https://doi.org/10.1007/978-3-030-28848-8_12

Cohen, O., Mahagna, A., Shamia, A., & Slobodin, O. (2020). Health-care services as a platform for building community resilience among minority communities: An Israeli pilot study during the COVID-19 outbreak. *International Journal of Environmental Research and Public Health, 17*(20), 7523. https://doi.org/10.3390/ijerph17207523

Counted, V. (2018). The Circle of Place Spirituality (CoPS): Towards an attachment and exploration motivational systems approach in the psychology of religion. In A. Village & R. W. Hood (Eds.), *Research in the social scientific study of religion* (Vol. 29, pp. 145–174). Brill. https://doi.org/10.1163/9789004382640_009

Counted, V., Neff, M. A., Captari, L. E., & Cowden, R. G. (2021). Transcending place attachment disruptions during a public health crisis: Spiritual struggles, resilience, and transformation. *Journal of Psychology and Christianity, 39*(4), 276–286.

Counted, V., & Zock, H. (2019). Place spirituality: An attachment perspective. *Archive for the Psychology of Religion, 41*(1), 12–25. https://doi.org/10.1177/0084672419833448

Devine-Wright, P., de Carvalho, L. P., Di Masso, A., Lewicka, M., Manzo, L., & Williams, D. R. (2020). "Re-placed"—Reconsidering relationships with place and lessons from a pandemic. *Journal of Environmental Psychology, 72*, 101514. https://doi.org/10.1016/j.jenvp.2020.101514

Fenton, A., Keegan, B., & Parry, K. (2020). Understanding sporting social media brand communities, place and social capital—A netnography of football fans. *Communication and Sport*. Advance online publication. https://doi.org/10.1177/2167479520986149

Guinart, D., & de Filippis, R. (2020). It's COVID o'clock—Time to publish or perish. *British Journal of Surgery, 108*(1), e44. https://doi.org/10.1093/bjs/znaa017

Huang, C., Huang, L., Wang, Y., Li, X., Ren, L., Gu, X., Kang, L., Guo, L., Liu, M., Zhou, X., Luo, J., Huang, Z., Tu, S., Zhao, Y., Chen, L., Xu, D., Li, Y., Li, C., Peng, L., ... Cao, B. (2021). 6-month consequences of COVID-19 in patients discharged from hospital: A cohort study. *Lancet, 397*(10270), 220–232. https://doi.org/10.1016/S0140-6736(20)32656-8

Kala, D. (2021). 'Thank you, God. You saved us'—Examining tourists' intention to visit religious destinations in the post COVID. *Current Issues in Tourism.* Advance online publication. https://doi.org/10.1080/13683500.2021.1876643

Kamata, H. (2021). Tourist destination residents' attitudes towards tourism during and after the COVID-19 pandemic. *Current Issues in Tourism.* Advance online publication. https://doi.org/10.1080/13683500.2021.1881452

Khalil, H., Peters, M., Godfrey, C. M., McInerney, P., Soares, C. B., & Parker, D. (2016). An evidence-based approach to scoping reviews. *Worldviews on Evidence-Based Nursing, 13*(2), 118–123. https://doi.org/10.1111/wvn.12144

Meagher, B. R., & Cheadle, A. D. (2020). Distant from others, but close to home: The relationship between home attachment and mental health during COVID-19. *Journal of Environmental Psychology, 72*, 101516. https://doi.org/10.1016/j.jenvp.2020.101516

Paköz, M. Z., Sözer, C., & Doğan, A. (2021). Changing perceptions and usage of public and pseudo-public spaces in the post-pandemic city: The case of Istanbul. *Urban Design International.* Advance online publication. https://doi.org/10.1057/s41289-020-00147-1

Parmar, A. (2020). Panic publishing: An unwarranted consequence of the COVID-19 pandemic. *Psychiatry Research, 294*, 113525. https://doi.org/10.1016/j.psychres.2020.113525

Peters, M. D. J., Godfrey, C., McInerney, P., Munn, Z., Tricco, A. C., & Khalil, H. (2020). Chapter 11: Scoping reviews. In E. Aromataris & Z. Munn (Eds.), *JBI manual for evidence synthesis.* Joanna Briggs Institute. https://doi.org/10.46658/JBIMES-20-12

Ramkissoon, H. (2020). COVID-19 Place confinement, pro-social, pro-environmental behaviors, and residents' wellbeing: A new conceptual framework. *Frontiers in Psychology, 11*, 2248. https://doi.org/10.3389/fpsyg.2020.02248

Scannell, L., & Gifford, R. (2017). Place attachment enhances psychological need satisfaction. *Environment and Behavior, 49*(4), 359–389. https://doi.org/10.1177/0013916516637648

Stieger, S., Lewetz, D., & Swami, V. (2021). Emotional well-being under conditions of lockdown: An experience sampling study in Austria during the COVID-19 pandemic. *Journal of Happiness Studies, 22*, 2703–2720. https://doi.org/10.1007/s10902-020-00337-2

Thompson-de Benoit, A., & Kramer, U. (2020). Work with emotions in remote psychotherapy in the time of Covid-19: A clinical experience. *Counselling Psychology Quarterly.* Advance online publication. https://doi.org/10.1080/09515070.2020.1770696

Tilaki, M. J. M., Abooali, G., Marzbali, M. H., & Samat, N. (2021). Vendors' attitudes and perceptions towards international tourists in the Malaysia night market: Does the COVID-19 outbreak matter? *Sustainability, 13*(3), 1553. https://doi.org/10.3390/su13031553

Tricco, A. C., Lillie, E., Zarin, W., O'Brien, K. K., Colquhoun, H., Levac, D., Moher, D., Peters, M., Horsley, T., Weeks, L., Hempel, S., Akl, E. A., Chang, C., McGowan, J., Stewart, L., Hartling, L., Aldcroft, A., Wilson, M. G., Garritty, C., ... Straus, S. E. (2018). PRISMA extension for scoping reviews (PRISMA-ScR): Checklist and explanation. *Annals of Internal Medicine, 169*(7), 467–473. https://doi.org/10.7326/M18-0850

Wang, F., Xue, T., Wang, T., & Wu, B. (2020). The mechanism of tourism risk perception in severe epidemic—The antecedent effect of place image depicted in anti-epidemic music videos and the moderating effect of visiting history. *Sustainability, 12*(13), 5454. https://doi.org/10.3390/su12135454

Chapter 3
Place Attachment and Resource Loss During a Pandemic: An Ecological Systems Perspective

Victor Counted, Richard G. Cowden, and Haywantee Ramkissoon

Contents

Conservation of Resources Theory and Principles.	34
Theory of Resource Loss.	34
Domains of Resource Loss.	34
Principles of Resource Loss.	34
Place Attachment Disruption and Resource Loss During the COVID-19 Pandemic: Separation from Significant Places and People in Place.	37
Place Attachment, Loss, and Recovery: Ecological Considerations During a Pandemic.	38
Ecological Propositions Associated with Place Attachment Disruption.	41
Proposition 1.	41
Proposition 2.	41
Proposition 3.	41
Proposition 4.	42
Conclusion.	42
References.	43

As we have learned from Bowlby's (1969) classic work on attachment and loss in Chapter 1 (see also Chapter 5), secure attachment relationships can support health and well-being. This attachment perspective lays the foundation for conceptualizing and understanding the emotional distress that may be experienced when place attachment disruption occurs. In this chapter, we discuss how the saliency of resource loss during the COVID-19 pandemic may have precipitated experiences of place attachment disruption. We also explore connections between the context of resource loss and social markers that can influence place attachment disruption, along with the implications of such disruption for increasing vulnerability to unfavorable economic, interpersonal, physical, and psychological outcomes.

Conservation of Resources Theory and Principles

Theory of Resource Loss

Hobfoll's (1988, 1989, 2001) conservation of resources (COR) theory provides us with a blueprint for exploring the cascading negative effects that disasters can have on health and well-being. Whereas other popular theories of stress (e.g., stress and coping theory; Lazarus & Folkman, 1984) tend to focus on how appraisal processes affect experiences of distress under challenging circumstances, COR theory emphasizes that stress arises when the demands of a particular situation outweigh the resources that a person has to offset those demands (Hobfoll et al., 2016). Hence, COR theory offers a guide for understanding how negative life events may precipitate resource loss and the dynamic consequences that unfold in response to disaster-related resource loss.

Domains of Resource Loss

According to COR theory (Hobfoll, 1988), resources are the experiences, objects, states, and conditions that people value. Hobfoll et al. (1995) noted four categories of resources that broadly meet our human needs, including (1) object resources (e.g., house, clothing), (2) personal resources (e.g., a sense of purpose, good health), (3) condition resources (e.g., job ranking, good relationship/marriage), and (4) energy resources (e.g., insurance, income). Although these are the general domains of resources that people value, there is no limit to what constitutes a resource (Hobfoll et al., 2016). The value of a specific resource can vary across individuals and cultures. A resource may be highly prized in one culture but have little value in another. This sort of relativism shapes what is considered a resource.

A basic tenet of COR theory is that people are naturally motivated to protect the resources they value (Hobfoll et al., 1995, 2016). Driven by this inherent survival mechanism, distress can arise when people are threatened with resource loss, actual resource loss occurs, or attempts to replace or substitute lost resources do not yield gains that are sufficient for offsetting resources that have been lost (see Chapter 6). In this chapter, we elaborate on the connections between these three scenarios and place attachment disruption within the context of the COVID-19 pandemic.

Principles of Resource Loss

COR theory posits four key principles of resource loss that provide a framework for understanding the dynamics that shape how people have been affected by resource loss during the public health crisis.

Principle 1: The Primacy of Loss The first principle states that resource loss is disproportionately more impactful than resource gain (Hobfoll et al., 2016). The loss of an object, condition, personal, or energy resource tends to be more detrimental to a person than if they were to gain the same resource. Resource loss tends to have a more pervasive effect, happens quickly, and impacts a person for a longer period than resource gain (Hobfoll et al., 2018). Loss of resources can become a threat to survival, especially when what might be lost in the process are resources that support one's existence.

There is strong support for the precedence of loss over gain within the cognitive psychology literature (Hobfoll et al., 2018; Mao et al., 2020), which has revealed that outcomes framed as loss tend to outweigh those framed in terms of resource gain. Research has shown that resource loss is strongly associated with psychological distress (Hobfoll et al., 1992, 2018), whereas the benefits of resource gains for alleviating psychological distress tends to be more limited (Hobfoll & Lilly, 1993). Resource gains that people accrue to offset resource loss within the context of the COVID-19 pandemic should not be overestimated, as the loss of valued resources have the potential to supersede resources that are gained (Cowden, Rueger, et al., 2021; Shammi et al., 2020).

Principle 2: Resource Investment This second principle of COR theory asserts that people must take steps to protect against the negative effects of resource loss by investing resources to regain, recover from, or compensate for what they have lost (Hobfoll et al., 2003, 2016). Resource investment can take the form of direct replacement of resources or resource substitution. Intentional attempts to replace or substitute lost resources can contribute to resource gains and facilitate recovery from resource loss (see Chapter 6).

Although resource loss in a time when multiple areas of human life have been severely affected may be particularly challenging to deal with, it is possible for people to cope and even thrive during the COVID-19 pandemic if the resources they invest offer some relief from what they have lost (Counted et al., 2020; see also Chapters 6 and 7). From a cognitive reframing perspective, resource investment could mean offsetting the loss of being separated from a place of attachment during the COVID-19 pandemic by reframing the situation more positively. For example, a person who has experienced place attachment disruption could reflect on their sense of connection to the broader environment that extends beyond any single place of attachment that has been disrupted by the public health crisis. Positive ambiances within a home could foster personal resources (e.g., sense of peace) that contribute to offsetting the loss of condition and energy resources among those who are emplaced in a home while adhering to strict stay-at-home orders (Meagher & Cheadle, 2020). When many tangible resources (i.e., income, job status) have been lost and there are few opportunities to recover those kinds of resources, it may be necessary to invest energy in immaterial resources (e.g., relationships, personal growth) that can support well-being over the short and long-term despite significant loss (Hobfoll et al., 2016; see also Chapter 7).

Principle 3: Gain Paradox COR theory also posits that conserving resources during a time of loss is paradoxical in that resource gain tends to become more salient when it transpires within the context of resource loss (Hobfoll et al., 2018). For example, finding hope may become a crucial personal resource during a disaster when tangible resources (e.g., income) have been lost, but it may not be as important when a person's system of existing resources is in balance. During the COVID-19 pandemic, many of the resources that were once available to people (e.g., jobs, financial stability) were lost, out of reach, or depleted. When resource loss occurs, it can spiral and lead to further losses (Hobfoll, 1998). Spirals of loss may be particularly devastating among people who are vulnerable to resource loss and those who have limited opportunities to gain resources. To limit the spiral of resource loss and initiate a process of recovery from losses, resource gain is necessary. The paradox of resource loss and gain is that spirals of each are complex, dynamic, and interdependent (Hobfoll et al., 2018). Loss cycles are usually more abrupt and potent than gain cycles, but spirals of resource gain can also follow a similar pattern in which gains in resources can lead to incremental and ongoing accumulation of resources (Hobfoll et al., 1995). Much like the potential long-term impact of resource loss, gains in resources can also have lasting implications for well-being. As people gain resources to offset pandemic-related resource loss, some may even build resources that promote well-being and facilitate resilience in response to future resource loss (see Chapter 6).

Principle 4: Desperation The fourth principle of COR theory is the notion of desperation (Hobfoll et al., 2018). This principle suggests that when people have exhausted their resources in the aftermath of a negative life event, they tend to enter a defensive, aggressive mode in which maladaptive behaviors become part of how they attempt to preserve the resources they value. Behaviors of desperation have not been uncommon during the COVID-19 pandemic. Many people publicly protested lockdown laws, calling it a *health dictatorship* (Smith, 2020). Some citizens referred to the public health restrictions as an *attack* on their personal freedom and a threat to their constitutional rights.

In Chapter 5, we discuss protest as a form of desperation response that can accompany a disrupted place attachment experience. People who are desperate to access places that they value may be at risk of severe distress (Counted et al., 2021). Desperation distress can be triggered by a number of factors tied to the COVID-19 pandemic. For example, desperation may arise from the frustration of being furloughed or retrenched because of the impact that widespread community mitigation strategies have had on business operations and the economy during the public health crisis. Protest behaviors that are rooted in desperation distress may continue until people find forms of resource investment that can effectively buffer the effects of losing access to places that are of significance to them.

Place Attachment Disruption and Resource Loss During the COVID-19 Pandemic: Separation from Significant Places and People in Place

One way of understanding how the COVID-19 pandemic has impacted our experiences with place is by considering intersections of place attachment and resource loss within the course of the public health crisis. First, the COVID-19 pandemic has affected the attachment bonds that people have with their cities, neighborhoods, school campuses, workplaces, and people within those places. These forms of place attachment disruption may have precipitated resource loss, which can lead to distress. Drawing on COR theory, stress can arise when a person is involuntarily separated from a place of attachment (see Chapter 6). Second, loss of resources during the public health crisis may have weakened the value of places within people's lives. For example, people may be less interested in traveling to destinations where the burden of COVID-19 is higher (Neuburger & Egger, 2021). Disrupted place attachment experiences during the COVID-19 pandemic have also limited our ability to access places (e.g., school campuses, workplaces) and people within places that are part of our daily routines (e.g., work colleagues, fellow students, community members). This disruption of place attachment can lead to a wide range of resource losses, which may contribute to a decreased sense of attachment to a place of significance.

Processing threat-related COVID-19 information may be the genesis of place attachment disruption. According to Bowlby's (1969) attachment theory, human beings are born with an innate psychological system, known as the attachment behavioral system, which drives them to seek proximity to attachment objects as a means of survival. This proximity-seeking behavior is a way of protecting the self from threats and dangers within the environment. When a person loses or is separated from an object of attachment, it can lead to an attachment disruption. Disruption in an attachment relationship occurs when there is a lack of emotional attunement, such that the individual is no longer able to recognize, understand, or engage with their object of attachment. The COVID-19 pandemic has threatened the perceived bond that many people have with significant attachment objects (e.g., places, people, God). For the purpose of this book, we are interested in how the public health crisis has threatened the bonds that people have with places that usually provide a sense of stability and continuity (e.g., school campuses, workplaces). The public health crisis has also disrupted our relationships with people in places where we work and live. The significant places (e.g., natural environment, cities, neighborhoods) and people in places (e.g., colleagues, friends, loved ones) that are part of our lives fall under the object resources domain (Hobfoll et al., 2018). Losing any of these object resources can become a disruptive process for those affected. Place attachment disruption may also elicit resource loss in the form of personal resource loss (e.g., diminished sense of security).

Several studies point to an increase in vulnerability to place attachment disruption during the COVID-19 pandemic (e.g., Ammar et al., 2020; Counted et al.,

2021; Stieger et al., 2021; Tscherning et al., 2020). If place attachment disruption manages to affect the availability of our resources by limiting our access to them, it could contribute to or exacerbate resource loss. Therefore, people must take necessary steps to protect these resources, especially in the context of a global public health crisis when resources may be under threat or in short supply (Counted et al., 2020; Govender et al., 2020). Place attachment is an essential resource for many people, and the conditions of the COVID-19 pandemic may have led people to adopt a defensive posture in order to protect this resource and deal with being separated from places of attachment.

When the places we are attached to and the people in those places are no longer available to us, a process of attachment disruption may ensue (Counted et al., 2021). We theorize that the first phase of place attachment disruption involves *protest*, followed by phases of *despair* and *detachment* (see Chapter 5). According to the Oxford dictionary, detachment is a "state of being objective or aloof." Thus, this phase of place attachment disruption could have positive or negative implications.

On the positive end of the spectrum, a person who is going through detachment could be objective and experience a positive shift in perspective. In contrast, detachment may be negative when it thrusts a person toward being alienated from their own thoughts and feelings. This maladaptive form of detachment may constitute a low level of emotional involvement with new experiences or relationships.

Ultimately, detachment reveals one of the great paradoxes of life. It teaches us that we must relinquish our former connections to recover from the loss we have experienced. Detachment also offers a lens that can be useful when thinking about post-pandemic recovery. That is, detachment has been theorized as a pathway for gaining more resources to sustain or enhance well-being in response to place attachment disruption that has transpired during the COVID-19 pandemic (Counted et al., 2021).

Place Attachment, Loss, and Recovery: Ecological Considerations During a Pandemic

Recovering from resource loss during a global pandemic, including those connected to places of attachment, requires people to invest in resources within the ecological contexts where they have been emplaced or displaced (Hobfoll et al., 1995). To understand how place attachment disruption related to resource loss may have impacted human life during the COVID-19 pandemic, we draw on an ecological framework of resource loss (Hobfoll et al., 1995). The ecological perspective sheds light on how the public health crisis has impacted resources that exist within the broad ecology of a person's life (see Fig. 3.1), including resources at organizational, community, family, and individual levels of society.

3 Place Attachment and Resource Loss During a Pandemic... 39

Resource loss at the organizational level will vary, as resources within this level often border the individual and family spheres (Hobfoll et al., 1995). For example, organizational resources can affect the availability of energy or condition resources. Many airline workers (e.g., pilots) and airport staff lost their jobs because governmental regulations resulted in a drastic reduction in air travel at different points during the public health disaster. The COVID-19 pandemic has also had devastating effects on the hospitality industry (Salem et al., 2021). As resorts, hotels, and other similar enterprises were forced to diminish operations, workers within the hospitality industry needed to reconsider their career options and find other sources of income. Due to the nature of their employment demands, healthcare workers and other essential workers have risked their own health and well-being by working on the front lines of the global pandemic. In vulnerable contexts where people often

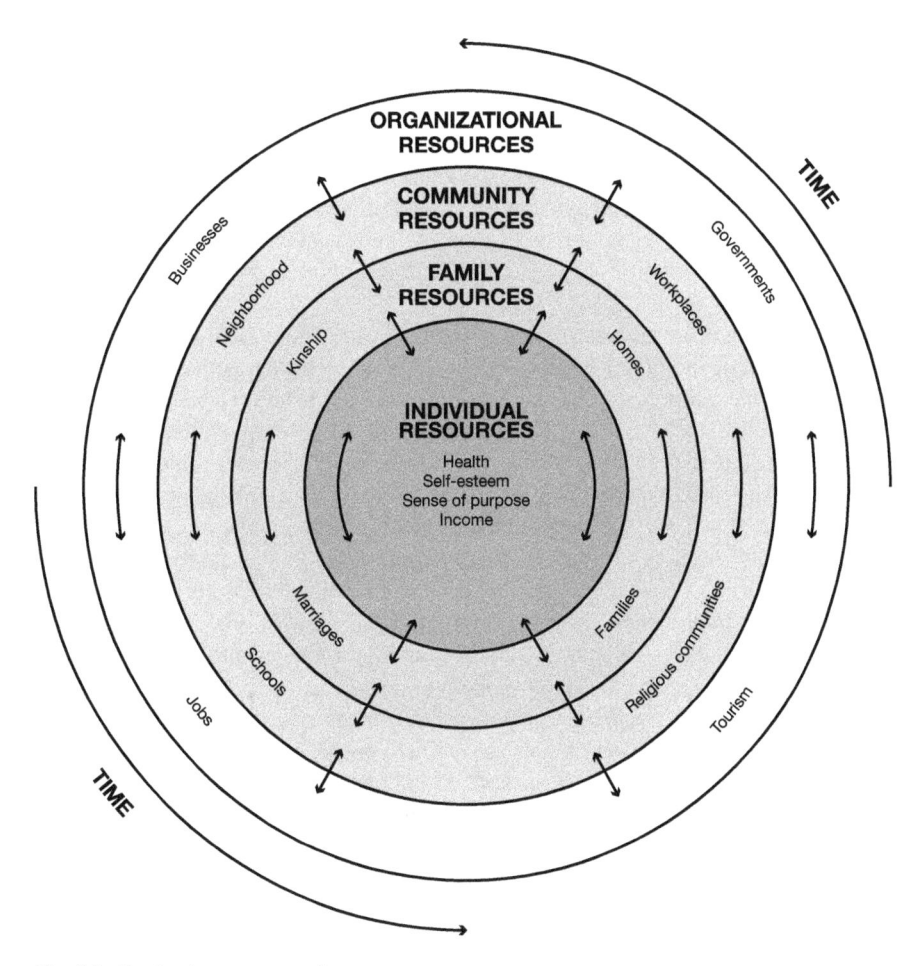

Fig. 3.1 Pandemic resource ecology

rely on organizational resources (e.g., nonprofit entities) to sustain themselves, people may have a particularly challenging time overcoming the loss of organizational resources (Govender et al., 2020).

The COVID-19 pandemic has also impacted resources that intersect the community level. School campuses or workplaces are examples of community-embedded object resources that many people have not been able to access during the public health crisis. Condition resources, such as the connections that a child values with other children in a neighborhood, have also been affected by how the public health crisis has changed local communities. However, resource loss can vary based on the context in which people live. In contexts where pervasive social-structural disadvantages exist, local communities may not have adequate resources to mitigate the community-level effects of the public health crisis on individual resources.

Resources that people value also intersect the family level, including condition (e.g., romantic partners) and object (e.g., family homes) resources. Some of these resources have been fractured by the COVID-19 pandemic. For example, the public health crisis seems to have become a catalyst for the separation and divorce of couples whose deep-seated relationship or marital issues have been unmasked by stay-at-home orders and other social distancing measures (Lebow, 2020). However, there are also narratives that highlight the gains in family resources that have transpired during the COVID-19 pandemic. For some people, romantic relationships with partners have strengthened and stay-at-home regulations have provided families with more opportunities to spend time with one another and develop more intimate connections (Milne et al., 2020).

Embedded within broader social systems are the individual-level condition, energy, personal, and object resources. The COVID-19 pandemic has had concerning implications for personal resources, such as mental health (Captari et al., 2021; Cowden, Davis, et al., 2021). Condition resources (e.g., employment) have been severely affected, with increasing reports of workers being furloughed or retrenched to manage the impact that the COVID-19 pandemic has had on businesses and other organizations (Fana et al., 2020). Such changes in condition resources also impact the availability of energy resources. For example, job loss has a direct effect on a person's financial well-being. Loss of resources within the course of the public health crisis will continue to have a profound negative effect on many individuals. Resource loss at organizational, community, and family levels may have long-term consequences for the availability of individual resources.

A person's entire ecological system of resources overlaps with place-based attachments, whether at a community level where people dwell and interact, organizational structures rooted in places of significance, or family and individual resources embedded within a geographical ensemble. Hence, resource loss that occurs during a global pandemic when widespread public health measures are implemented to protect human lives can be considered a place-based event.

Ecological Propositions Associated with Place Attachment Disruption

COR theory emphasizes the importance of understanding people as those who possess many individual resources, share some family and community resources, and have possible access to organizational resources within a social system (see Fig. 3.1). The ecological model of resource loss illustrates how a global pandemic can affect condition, energy, object, and personal resources at different levels of the ecological system, ranging from the individual level through to the organizational level. Using this ecological framework, we outline propositions about how people-place relationships might be affected by a pandemic.

Proposition 1

Resource loss will have its strongest impact on resources at the individual and family levels when a pandemic disrupts relationships with place because they are proximal and the first to be impacted. According to the gain paradox of COR theory, resource loss cycles are potent and tend to have a more immediate effect on proximal resources, which can lead to spirals of loss that extend to other areas of human life. For example, place attachment disruption during a pandemic could have debilitating effects on individual resources (e.g., life balance). Over time, loss of individual resources could impact the availability of resources at more distal levels (e.g., family resources).

Proposition 2

Resource loss that accompanies attachment disruption during a pandemic may inhibit people from effectively coping with its impact on their family and individual resources. For example, if community-level resources are limited because people have been unable to access places of attachment during a pandemic, it will also detract from the availability of family and individual resources.

Proposition 3

When place attachment disruption occurs, the loss of a resource at one level (e.g., family) may be compensated for by resources at other levels (e.g., organizational level). However, loss of certain resources may be difficult for people to offset because of how they overlap with different ecological levels. Hobfoll et al. (1995)

describe this phenomenon as *border resources*, which refers to the idea that "individual and family spheres may be joined at their borders with the organizational and community spheres" (p. 44). Place attachment tends to be a border resource because it intersects with multiple levels of ecology. For example, both personal (e.g., spiritual well-being) and community resources (e.g., social support) are accessed and cultivated in places of worship that are sacred to many people. However, the implication of border resources is that disruption of such resources can affect the availability of resources at other levels within an ecological system (Hobfoll et al., 1995, 2016), which suggests that it may be particularly important to protect and conserve a border resource like place attachment.

Proposition 4

Overlapping to some extent with proposition three, the fourth proposition reveals the limitations of border resources during a place attachment disruption. Hobfoll et al. (1995) reasoned that border resource loss is "a disassociation of the individual from the family, the family from the organization, or the organization from the community" (p. 44). When the *connective fabric* that binds the different systems of resources is disintegrated along with the disrupted place attachment, cross-border resource utilization is impaired and vulnerability to ongoing resource loss is increased (Hobfoll et al., 2016). Hence, we propose that people will lose their capacity to benefit from an integrated arrangement of resources when border resources are lost during an experience of place attachment disruption.

Conclusion

COR theory reminds us that people are susceptible to the stress of resource loss in times of crisis. In this chapter, we discussed the intricacies and interrelationships between resource loss and place attachment disruption within the context of a global pandemic. By highlighting how place attachment disruption can contribute to resource loss and widen the pre-existing systemic vulnerabilities that impact individual, family, community, and organizational levels of a person's ecological system, we hope that this perspective provides a framework that place scholars can use in their work. The resource ecology framework could help us to identify where pandemic-related losses have occurred within our society and how to address the mechanisms by which place attachment disruption leads to resource loss. Resource investment at different levels of society will be critical for promoting recovery within the larger ecological system, both during and after global health crises such as the COVID-19 pandemic.

References

Ammar, A., Mueller, P., Trabelsi, K., Chtourou, H., Boukhris, O., Masmoudi, L., Bouaziz, B., Brach, M., Schmicker, M., Bentlage, E., How, D., Ahmed, M., Aloui, A., Hammouda, O., Paineiras-Domingos, L. L., Braakman-jansen, A., Wrede, C., Bastoni, S., Pernambuco, C. S., ..., ECLB-COVID19 Consortium. (2020). Psychological consequences of COVID-19 home confinement: The ECLB-COVID19 multicenter study. *PLoS One, 15*(11), e0240204. https://doi.org/10.1371/journal.pone.0240204.

Bowlby, J. (1969). *Attachment and loss: Attachment* (Vol. 1). Basic Books.

Captari, L. E., Cowden, R. G., Davis, E. B., Standage, S., & Counted, V. (2021). *Religious/spiritual struggles and depression during COVID-19 pandemic lockdowns in the Global South: Evidence of moderation by positive religious coping and hope*. Manuscript submitted for publication.

Counted, V., Neff, M. A., Captari, L. E., & Cowden, R. G. (2021). Transcending place attachment disruptions during a public health crisis: Spiritual struggles, resilience, and transformation. *Journal of Psychology and Christianity, 39*(4), 276–286.

Counted, V., Pargament, K. I., Bachera, A. O., Joynt, S., & Cowden, R. G. (2020). Hope and well-being in vulnerable contexts during the COVID-19 pandemic: Does religious coping matter? *The Journal of Positive Psychology*. Advance online publication. https://doi.org/10.1080/17439760.2020.1832247

Cowden, R. G., Davis, E. B., Counted, V., Chen, Y., Rueger, S. Y., VanderWeele, T. J., Lemke, A. W., Glowiak, K. J., & Worthington, E. L., Jr. (2021). Suffering, mental health, and psychological well-being during the COVID-19 pandemic: A longitudinal study of U.S. adults with chronic health conditions. *Wellbeing, Space and Society, 2*, 100048. https://doi.org/10.1016/j.wss.2021.100048

Cowden, R. G., Rueger, S. Y., Davis, E. B., Counted, V., Kent, B. V., Chen, Y., VanderWeele, T. J., Rim, M., Lemke, A. W., & Worthington, E. L., Jr. (2021). Resource loss, positive religious coping, and suffering during the COVID-19 pandemic: A prospective cohort study of U.S. adults with chronic illness. *Mental Health, Religion & Culture*. Advance online publication. https://doi.org/10.1080/13674676.2021.1948000

Fana, M., Torrejón Pérez, S., & Fernández-Macías, E. (2020). Employment impact of Covid-19 crisis: From short term effects to long terms prospects. *Journal of Industrial and Business Economics, 47*, 391–410. https://doi.org/10.1007/s40812-020-00168-5

Govender, K., Cowden, R. G., Nyamaruze, P., Armstrong, R. M., & Hatane, L. (2020). Beyond the disease: Contextualized implications of the COVID-19 pandemic for children and young people living in Eastern and Southern Africa. *Frontiers in Public Health, 8*, 504. https://doi.org/10.3389/fpubh.2020.00504

Hobfoll, S. E. (1988). *The ecology of stress*. Hemisphere Publishing Corp.

Hobfoll, S. E. (1989). Conservation of resources: A new attempt at conceptualizing stress. *American Psychologist, 44*(3), 513–524. https://doi.org/10.1037//0003-066x.44.3.513

Hobfoll, S. E. (1998). *Stress, culture, and community: The psychology and philosophy of stress*. Plenum Press.

Hobfoll, S. E. (2001). The influence of culture, community, and the nested-self in the stress process: Advancing conservation of resources theory. *Applied Psychology, 50*(3), 337–421. https://doi.org/10.1111/1464-0597.00062

Hobfoll, S. E., Dunahoo, C. A., & Monnier, J. (1995). Conservation of resources and traumatic stress. In S. E. Hobfoll & J. R. Freedy (Eds.), *Traumatic stress: From theory to practice* (pp. 29–47). Plenum Press. https://doi.org/10.1007/978-1-4899-1076-9_2

Hobfoll, S. E., Halbesleben, J., Neveu, J. P., & Westman, M. (2018). Conservation of resources in the organizational context: The reality of resources and their consequences. *Annual Review of Organizational Psychology and Organizational Behavior, 5*(1), 103–128. https://doi.org/10.1146/annurev-orgpsych-032117-104640

Hobfoll, S. E., Johnson, R. J., Ennis, N., & Jackson, A. P. (2003). Resource loss, resource gain, and emotional outcomes among inner city women. *Journal of Personality and Social Psychology, 84*(3), 632–643. https://doi.org/10.1037/0022-3514.84.3.632

Hobfoll, S. E., & Lilly, R. S. (1993). Resource conservation as a strategy for community psychology. *Journal of Community Psychology, 21*(2), 128–148. https://doi.org/10.1002/1520-6629(199304)21:2%3C128::AID-JCOP2290210206%3E3.0.CO;2-5

Hobfoll, S. E., Lilly, R. S., & Jackson, A. P. (1992). Conservation of social resources and the self. In H. O. F. Veiel & U. Baumann (Eds.), *The meaning and measurement of social support* (pp. 125–141). Hemisphere Publishing Corp.

Hobfoll, S. E., Tirone, V., Holmgreen, L., & Gerhart, J. (2016). Conservation of resources theory applied to major stress. In G. Fink (Ed.), *Stress: Concepts, cognition, emotion, and behavior* (pp. 65–71). Academic. https://doi.org/10.1016/B978-0-12-800951-2.00007-8

Lazarus, R. S., & Folkman, S. (1984). *Stress, appraisal, and coping*. Springer.

Lebow, J. L. (2020). The challenges of COVID-19 for divorcing and post-divorce families. *Family Process, 59*(3), 967–973. https://doi.org/10.1111/famp.12574

Mao, Y., He, J., Morrison, A. M., & Coca-Stefaniak, J. A. (2020). Effects of tourism CSR on employee psychological capital in the COVID-19 crisis: From the perspective of conservation of resources theory. *Current Issues in Tourism*. Advance online publication. https://doi.org/10.1080/13683500.2020.1770706

Meagher, B. R., & Cheadle, A. D. (2020). Distant from others, but close to home: The relationship between home attachment and mental health during COVID-19. *Journal of Environmental Psychology, 72*, 101516. https://doi.org/10.1016/j.jenvp.2020.101516

Milne, S. J., Corbett, G. A., Hehir, M. P., Lindow, S. W., Mohan, S., Reagu, S., Farrell, T., & O'Connell, M. P. (2020). Effects of isolation on mood and relationships in pregnant women during the covid-19 pandemic. *European Journal of Obstetrics, Gynecology, and Reproductive Biology, 252*, 610–611. https://doi.org/10.1016/j.ejogrb.2020.06.009

Neuburger, L., & Egger, R. (2021). Travel risk perception and travel behaviour during the COVID-19 pandemic 2020: A case study of the DACH region. *Current Issues in Tourism, 24*(7), 1003–1016. https://doi.org/10.1080/13683500.2020.1803807

Salem, I. E., Elkhwesky, Z., & Ramkissoon, H. (2021). A content analysis for government's and hotels' response to COVID-19 pandemic in Egypt. *Tourism and Hospitality Research*. Advance online publication. https://doi.org/10.1177/14673584211002614

Shammi, M., Bodrud-Doza, M., Islam, A. R. M. T., & Rahman, M. M. (2020). COVID-19 pandemic, socioeconomic crisis and human stress in resource-limited settings: A case from Bangladesh. *Heliyon, 6*(5), e04063. https://doi.org/10.1016/j.heliyon.2020.e04063

Smith, P. (2020). Hard lockdown and a "health dictatorship": Australia's lucky escape from covid-19. *BMJ, 371*, m4910. https://doi.org/10.1136/bmj.m4910

Stieger, S., Lewetz, D., & Swami, V. (2021). Emotional well-being under conditions of lockdown: An experience sampling study in Austria during the COVID-19 pandemic. *Journal of Happiness Studies, 22*, 2703–2720. https://doi.org/10.1007/s10902-020-00337-2

Tscherning, C., Sizun, J., & Kuhn, P. (2020). Promoting attachment between parents and neonates despite the COVID-19 pandemic. *Acta Paediatrica, 109*(10), 1937–1943. https://doi.org/10.1111/apa.15455

Chapter 4
Place Attachment and Suffering During a Pandemic

Richard G. Cowden, Victor Counted, and Haywantee Ramkissoon

Contents

Revisiting People-Place Relationships and Place Attachment Disruption	46
Background on Suffering	47
Place Attachment Disruption and Suffering	49
Conclusion	51
References	52

Since the SARS-CoV-2 outbreak emerged in late 2019, loss has been part of the individual and collective experiences of people all over the world. Of principal concern has been the loss of life. At the time of writing, more than 2.5 million COVID-19 deaths had been reported worldwide since the first case of SARS-CoV-2 was confirmed (World Health Organization, 2021). However, the devastating health impact of COVID-19 has occurred in parallel with numerous other losses (Cowden, Davis, et al., 2021; Cowden, Rueger, et al., 2021).

To prevent excess mortality and healthcare systems from being overwhelmed (Govender et al., 2020), government authorities in many parts of the world implemented community mitigation strategies to prevent or reduce transmission of SARS-CoV-2. Although public health control measures centered on limiting person-to-person contact, varying degrees of restrictions were imposed. Several countries and territories implemented stringent lockdowns at one time or another (Chaudhry et al., 2020), which have generally included some combination of stay-at-home orders, bans on long-distance travel (both locally and internationally), cancellation of mass social gatherings, and suspension of non-essential in-person operations of businesses and other institutions (e.g., educational establishments, faith-based organizations). Citizens of some countries were initially subjected to a single, strict lockdown that was gradually eased over time (e.g., South Africa), whereas others have experienced fluctuating levels of more versus less restrictive lockdowns over the course of several months (e.g., Philippines).

The secondary losses that have accompanied community mitigation strategies during the COVID-19 pandemic, particularly those involving lockdowns, are numerous. For example, people have lost their former routines of daily life, in-person contact with social support networks, and community-based activities (e.g., religious services) that were a prominent part of their lives (Counted et al., 2020; Marroquín et al., 2020; VanderWeele, 2020; van Tilburg et al., 2020). Many of these losses are tethered to place attachment disruptions that public health control measures have precipitated, the consequences of which could impact negatively on psychological, social, and spiritual well-being (Counted et al., 2021). This chapter discusses the potential for pandemic-related disruptions to the bonds that people have with places, along with secondary losses connected to those disrupted place attachments, to evoke a state of suffering.

Revisiting People-Place Relationships and Place Attachment Disruption

The concept of place refers to any valued environmental space that carries meaning (Sime, 1986). In environmental psychology, various place-based concepts (e.g., place attachment, place-identity, geographic ensemble, genius loci, place dependence, people in place, sense of community, sense of place) have emerged to account for the intricate way in which well-being might be influenced through one's association with the environment (Peng et al., 2020). The focus of this chapter will be on place attachment, because it is particularly relevant to understanding the impact that separation from a place of significance could have on suffering.

Places function as relational objects to which relationships are formed (Counted et al., 2021; Jorgensen & Stedman, 2001). Through personal experience with the environment, people develop connections to places (Clarke et al., 2018). Although people-place relationships ordinarily involve some level of connection to the concrete spatial features of a location, people-place relationships are intricately connected to a broader range of intrapersonal (e.g., self-identity), interpersonal (e.g., social connection), and transcendental (e.g., spirituality) phenomena (Counted, 2018; Lewicka, 2011). A broad term commonly used to describe the bonds that people develop with various places is place attachment (Hidalgo & Hernández, 2001).

Place attachment functions similarly to other significant objects of attachment (Counted et al., 2021). Studies have found that places of attachment can be experienced as a sanctum, giving people a sense of comfort, security, and stability (Scannell & Gifford, 2010). Place attachment can also foster belongingness by sustaining symbolic connections to cultural history and family heritage (Captari et al., 2019; Li & Chan, 2018). Some evidence suggests that place attachment supports self-regulatory processes (e.g., self-reflection) that facilitate personal growth (Scannell & Gifford, 2017). For some people, places of attachment restore psychological balance by cultivating positive emotions and relieving stress (Korpela, 2012). Together, these benefits of place attachment highlight how people's bonds with places can serve as a resource for supporting well-being. When access to that resource is disrupted, it can have negative implications for well-being.

Place attachment disruption occurs when people are separated from a place that holds significance (Scannell et al., 2021). That experience can be devastating, as place attachment disruption typically brings about many other types of losses (Scannell et al., 2016). Losses that are precipitated by place attachment disruption can challenge various aspects of a person's general orienting system, a broad term that refers to how a person typically views, makes sense of, and relates to the world (Pargament, 2001). Studies have revealed that place attachment disruption undermines identity continuity. People sometimes find it difficult to re-establish a sense of stability or recover a positive identity following disruption to the bond they have with a place (Brown & Perkins, 1992). Place attachment disruption may also be corrosive to a person's relational well-being because places of attachment often serve as contexts for people to build and strengthen social bonds (Scannell & Gifford, 2017). When place attachment disruption involves a sacred space, it can interfere with religious/spiritual experiences (e.g., closeness to the divine, life cycle rituals) and faith-based community ties that enrich a person's religious/spiritual self (Captari et al., 2019; Counted et al., 2021; Mazumdar & Mazumdar, 2004). These consequences of place attachment disruption reveal some of the ways it may affect a person's orienting system, which can lead to distress (Scannell et al., 2016). Under certain conditions, the distress that accompanies place attachment disruption might constitute suffering.

Background on Suffering

The concept of suffering has received considerable attention from many philosophical and religious traditions that have attempted to clarify its nature, meaning, and implications for well-being. Some historical descriptions highlight the pernicious impact that suffering can have on well-being. In *Nicomachean Ethics*, Aristotle (1999) uses King Priam's grief over the death of his son to illustrate how suffering may prevent even the most noble and virtuous of people from reaching a state of complete happiness. Other perspectives portray a more subtle and pervasive kind of suffering that lingers almost constantly throughout a person's life. Schopenhauer (1909) posits that all suffering originates from desires of "the will." Desires are impossible to permanently satisfy because an infinite number of human desires exist, and each one that is fulfilled ordinarily gives rise to a new one. From this perspective, suffering is a routine and unavoidable part of being human.

In other descriptions, the inevitability of suffering is acknowledged, but the principal focus is on the meaning of suffering. John Paul II (1984) describes suffering as *salvific*, emphasizing the capacity for suffering to be redeemed for a higher purpose. A transcendent and transformational view of suffering can also be found in the writings of other religious traditions. In Hinduism, suffering (by way of *karma*) presents an opportunity to be tested, learn, and grow on one's spiritual journey to transcendence (Whitman, 2007). Within the Islamic tradition (and to some extent Christianity), suffering serves an instrumental function as part of the divine's plan to bring one closer to God and self-actualization (Mobin-Uddin, 2018). Although far from an exhaustive account of the philosophical and religious perspectives on suffering, they broadly sketch the long-standing interest humanity has had in understanding the enigma of suffering and the complexity of its connection to the human condition.

Suffering might be understood as a negatively valenced subjective state that involves bearing under loss or privation of some perceived good (VanderWeele, 2019). It is entangled in the very essence of human existence, and it is an experience that tends to become more familiar the longer one lives. Although there is a universal component to suffering, the experience itself is personal, complex, and dynamic (Cassell, 1999). People interpret, label, and make sense of phenomena through a person-specific meaning-making lens that is shaped over time by a combination of biological, physical, cultural, spiritual, and relational experiences (Cassell, 1982; Fitzpatrick et al., 2016). This personalized lens influences the content and valence of phenomenological experiences, including those concerning suffering. Two people may be confronted with the same loss (e.g., disruption to place attachment), but experiences of suffering may vary considerably (Tate & Pearlman, 2019). The potential also exists for first-person experiences of suffering to shift (positively or negatively), even if a person's circumstances remain unchanged. A positive reinterpretation of one's circumstances may alleviate suffering, whereas a more pronounced focus on the negative aspects of one's experience may exacerbate suffering.

Suffering has most commonly been applied to develop a more complete understanding of the subjective experiences of distress among people who have physical pain, illness, or symptoms (Cowden, Davis, et al., 2021). However, suffering can originate from a broad range of domains that extend beyond the boundaries of physical health, including psychological (e.g., mental health problems), relational (e.g., social disconnection), spiritual (e.g., spiritual discontent), and systemic (e.g., poverty) causes. Moreover, the cause and object of suffering may be distinct (VanderWeele, 2019). Place attachment disruption during the COVID-19 pandemic may be the principal cause of a person's suffering, but the object of their suffering might be an acute sense of identity loss.

The concept of suffering is multifaceted. Suffering usually involves some level of perceived intolerability concerning the intensity of the negative experience or length of time one expects the undesired state to last (VanderWeele, 2019). It may evolve from an isolated secondary concern to become a primary source of distress that permeates all aspects of a person's life (Cassell, 2004). Such a corrosive process can threaten one's personhood by fracturing social relationships, disrupting life purposes, and shaking previously held beliefs about the world (Tate & Pearlman, 2019). Suffering also entails some sense of powerlessness over the extent or duration of one's suffering (VanderWeele, 2019). An event or action that precipitated one's state of suffering may have been within a person's control, but one may be unable to control the experience of suffering itself.

Place Attachment Disruption and Suffering

A variety of place attachment disruptions have transpired during the COVID-19 pandemic. Some have been uncommon (e.g., involuntary emplacement abroad due to border closures), whereas others have been shared by many people around the world (e.g., closure of places of worship). The most sweeping forms of place attachment disruption have originated from community mitigation strategies (e.g., social distancing). Access to places of attachment that routinely form part of daily life (e.g., workplaces, schools) has been limited, many of which serve important functions in supporting well-being (Scannell & Gifford, 2016, 2017). When restrictions concerning access to spaces are relaxed or lifted, the positive undertones associated with many places of attachment could be met with undesirable concerns about acquisition and transmission of SARS-CoV-2 (Counted et al., 2021). Other forms of place attachment disruption amid the public health crisis have had a greater impact on specific individuals or groups of people. At times, traditional forms of religious/spiritual rituals, ceremonies, and commemorative events have been unfeasible or prohibited. Rites of passage (e.g., funerals) have been modified to conform to public health measures, including those customarily performed in places of significance (Hamid & Jahangir, 2020).

Although place attachment disruptions during the COVID-19 pandemic have been ubiquitous, experiences of place attachment disruption are connected to the broader context in which people live. In states and territories where stringent stay-at-home orders were imposed (e.g., South Africa, United Kingdom), people were largely confined to the boundaries of their homes (Ramkissoon, 2020). For people living in contexts of social-structural disadvantage, strict emplacement might have exacerbated pre-existing challenges (e.g., food insecurity) and deprived people of access to resources (e.g., social support) that are often tethered to places of attachment (Counted et al., 2021).

When place attachment disruption is prolonged or remains unrepaired, a person may be vulnerable to a persistent state of distress that constitutes suffering. One useful framework for understanding how suffering might arise from pandemic-related place attachment disruption is the *Four Noble Truths*, a set of Buddhist teachings on suffering and impermanence (Asaṅga, 2001). The first noble truth, *dukkha*, addresses the existence of suffering. Its meaning reflects a continuum of suffering ranging from a level of dissatisfaction that is barely noticeable to a state of extreme suffering (Anālayo, 2013). This conception of suffering tends to be more encompassing than conventional Western perspectives (Van Gordon et al., 2015), but this does not imply that all suffering is the same. Three superordinate forms of suffering are captured under the banner of dukkha, each of which is rooted in the transformation and impermanence that embodies human existence (Asaṅga, 2001).

The most subtle form of suffering is *saṅkhāra dukkha* ("suffering of conditioned existence"), which is a mysterious kind of suffering that is all-pervasive (Chang, 2019). It emanates from a fixed or ignorant perception of the ever-changing nature of our psychophysical experience (Van Gordon et al., 2015). According to Buddhist thought, this distorted perception of reality is not fully appreciable by the average person. Sensitization of the mind to this source of dissatisfaction is said to bring one closer to *enlightenment* (Walsh, 1995). Although saṅkhāra dukkha is an important part of understanding the Buddhist conception of suffering as an enduring latent state that permeates throughout the course of one's life (Van Gordon et al., 2015), the two more tangible forms of dukkha are particularly useful for appreciating experiences of suffering that might arise from place disruption during the COVID-19 pandemic.

Vipariṇāma dukkha ("suffering of transformation") can be found in any phenomenon that is temporary or subject to change (Chang, 2019). It is reflected in the near-constant unsatisfactoriness inherent in the change, ambiguity, and impermanence that characterizes human existence (Walsh, 1995). Although suffering of transformation originates from change (Asaṅga, 2001), it is revealed in our resistance or inability to accept change (Teasdale & Chaskalson, 2011). Place attachment disruption is a change that is challenging to accept because people-place bonds usually develop slowly over time, disruptions to place usually underlie other ancillary changes, and people are forced to deal with such change without being able to access the suite of place-based resources that could support adjustment to change (Brown & Perkins, 1992; Scannell et al., 2016). During the COVID-19 pandemic, many people have encountered changes linked to involuntary separation from places of attachment. Given the evolving nature of the public health crisis, those who attempt to "hold" onto their places of attachment might be more vulnerable to a subjective state of suffering.

The most palpable form of suffering in Buddhism is *dukkha dukkha* ("suffering of suffering"). It commonly refers to the physically or psychologically agonizing experiences that accompany difficult transitions in life (e.g., illness, loss of life), but more broadly encompasses having to endure situations that are deemed unpleasant (Asaṅga, 2001; Chang, 2019). Mentally or physically painful experiences in themselves do not necessarily constitute dukkha dukkha, but rather it is the mental processes which follow such experiences (e.g., ruminative thinking) that lead to a state of suffering (Teasdale & Chaskalson, 2011). This form of suffering resonates closely with the notion that place attachment disruption is a characteristically unpleasant experience (Scannell et al., 2016; Scannell & Gifford, 2017).

Many people may describe the unpleasantness of their pandemic-related place attachment disruption experience in a way that is consistent with suffering. People all over the world have been unable to access places of attachment at one time or another. Separation from a place of attachment within the course of the public health crisis might constitute or be accompanied by the loss of some perceived good. Pandemic-related place attachment disruption may be the principal cause of a person's suffering, but the object of suffering could also comprise any number of secondary losses (e.g., life balance, sense of peace) which might be tethered to the place of attachment that has been disrupted by conditions of the COVID-19 pandemic. Suffering that is associated with separation from places of attachment during the COVID-19 pandemic may pose a threat to different aspects of one's personhood, such as one's understanding of the world, social relationships, or religious/

spiritual life. The findings of several studies that have been conducted outside the context of the COVID-19 pandemic suggest that perceived disruption to place attachment can affect the intactness of a person (Boğaç, 2009; Brown & Perkins, 1992; Scannell & Gifford, 2017).

Another feature of the public health crisis that could precipitate suffering in the aftermath of place attachment disruption is its ambiguous timeline. In certain countries (e.g., Colombia), lockdowns were extended on multiple occasions. Other communities were subjected to phases in which public health measures were imposed, relaxed, and re-instated intermittently. These kinds of uncertainties could affect the outlook that people have about the duration they expect to endure public health control measures. If reasonable opportunities to reunite with places of attachment seem improbable in the near future, some people may anticipate needing to endure the losses that arise from place attachment disruption for a length of time that feels unbearable. Moreover, community mitigation strategies were essentially implemented and regulated by government authorities (Counted et al., 2021). Thus, people had limited control over the duration they had to endure that which had been lost due to place attachment disruption. That sense of powerlessness could exacerbate experiences of suffering.

Place attachment disruption experiences may be distressing, but suffering is not an inevitable state for people who have been confronted with pandemic-related disruption. Even when place attachment disruption leads to a subjective state of suffering, the consequences of suffering may not be wholly objectionable. Suffering indicates to a person that whatever has been lost needs to be adjusted to, compensated for, or regained (VanderWeele, 2019). That signal can serve an adaptive function in prompting constructive responses that facilitate adjustment and personal growth. One possible response is *detachment* behavior (Counted et al., 2021; see also Chapter 5), which involves finding new forms of relationships outside of the place of attachment (e.g., turning to the sacred for relationship). Other psychospiritual processes (e.g., meaning-making, mindfulness) may also assist people with transcending suffering that is attributable to pandemic-related place attachment disruption.

Conclusion

The COVID-19 pandemic has been a common cause of place attachment disruption for people in almost every part of the world. Place attachment disruption is often accompanied by distress (Scannell et al., 2016), and yet the subjective experiences of people who have been separated from places of attachment can vary considerably (Boğaç, 2009; Brown & Perkins, 1992). Just as the public health crisis has forced humanity to re-evaluate some of its most widely held assumptions about the world (e.g., perceived sense of control), it has also exposed a need to develop an improved understanding of how people experience and respond to place attachment disruption. By exploring the potential for pandemic-related place attachment disruption to elicit a state of distress that constitutes suffering, this chapter has drawn attention to the complex subjective experiences of people who have been separated from places of attachment. Although the concept of suffering may not apply to all people who have experienced pandemic-related place attachment disruption, it may contribute to building a richer understanding of the implications of place attachment disruption for well-being. That could lead to more informed treatment approaches for supporting people who have been separated from places of attachment, both during the COVID-19 pandemic and in time to come.

References

Anālayo, B. (2013). Dukkha. In A. L. C. Runehov & L. Oviedo (Eds.), *Encyclopedia of sciences and religions* (pp. 647–649). Springer. https://doi.org/10.1007/978-1-4020-8265-8_1616
Aristotle. (1999). *Nicomachean ethics* (W. D. Ross, Trans.). Batoche Books.
Asaṅga. (2001). *Abhidharmasamuccaya: The compendium of higher teaching (philosophy)*. Jain Publishing Company.
Boğaç, C. (2009). Place attachment in a foreign settlement. *Journal of Environmental Psychology, 29*(2), 267–278. https://doi.org/10.1016/j.jenvp.2009.01.001
Brown, B. B., & Perkins, D. D. (1992). Disruptions in place attachment. In I. Altman & S. M. Low (Eds.), *Place attachment* (pp. 279–304). Springer. https://doi.org/10.1007/978-1-4684-8753-4_13
Captari, L. E., Hook, J. N., Aten, J. D., Davis, E. B., & Tisdale, T. C. (2019). Embodied spirituality following disaster: Exploring intersections of religious and place attachment in resilience and meaning-making. In V. Counted & F. Watts (Eds.), *The psychology of religion and place* (pp. 49–79). Palgrave Macmillan. https://doi.org/10.1007/978-3-030-28848-8_4
Cassell, E. J. (1982). The nature of suffering and the goals of medicine. *The New England Journal of Medicine, 306*(11), 639–645. https://doi.org/10.1056/NEJM198203183061104
Cassell, E. J. (1999). Diagnosing suffering: A perspective. *Annals of Internal Medicine, 131*(7), 531–534. https://doi.org/10.7326/0003-4819-131-7-199910050-00009
Cassell, E. J. (2004). *The nature of suffering and the goals of medicine* (2nd ed.). Oxford University Press.
Chang, A. (2019). The gerontology of suffering and its social remediation: A Buddhist perspective. *Journal of Religion, Spirituality & Aging, 31*(4), 400–413. https://doi.org/10.1080/15528030.2018.1550733
Chaudhry, R., Dranitsaris, G., Mubashir, T., Bartoszko, J., & Riazi, S. (2020). A country level analysis measuring the impact of government actions, country preparedness and socioeconomic factors on COVID-19 mortality and related health outcomes. *EClinicalMedicine, 25*, 100464. https://doi.org/10.1016/j.eclinm.2020.100464
Clarke, D., Murphy, C., & Lorenzoni, I. (2018). Place attachment, disruption and transformative adaptation. *Journal of Environmental Psychology, 55*, 81–89. https://doi.org/10.1016/j.jenvp.2017.12.006
Counted, V. (2018). The Circle of Place Spirituality (CoPS): Towards an attachment and exploration motivational systems approach in the psychology of religion. In A. Village & R. W. Hood (Eds.), *Research in the social scientific study of religion* (Vol. 29, pp. 145–174). Brill. https://doi.org/10.1163/9789004382640_009
Counted, V., Neff, M. A., Captari, L. E., & Cowden, R. G. (2021). Transcending place attachment disruptions during a public health crisis: Spiritual struggles, resilience, and transformation. *Journal of Psychology and Christianity, 39*(4), 276–286.

Counted, V., Pargament, K. I., Bechara, A. O., Joynt, S., & Cowden, R. G. (2020). Hope and well-being in vulnerable contexts during the COVID-19 pandemic: Does religious coping matter? *The Journal of Positive Psychology*. Advance online publication. https://doi.org/10.1080/17439760.2020.1832247

Cowden, R. G., Davis, E. B., Counted, V., Chen, Y., Rueger, S. Y., VanderWeele, T. J., Lemke, A. W., Glowiak, K. J., & Worthington, E. L., Jr. (2021). Suffering, mental health, and psychological well-being during the COVID-19 pandemic: A longitudinal study of U.S. adults with chronic health conditions. *Wellbeing, Space and Society, 2*, 100048. https://doi.org/10.1016/j.wss.2021.100048

Cowden, R. G., Rueger, S. Y., Davis, E. B., Counted, V., Kent, B. V., Chen, Y., VanderWeele, T. J., Rim, M., Lemke, A. W., & Worthington, E. L., Jr. (2021). Resource loss, positive religious coping, and suffering during the COVID-19 pandemic: A prospective cohort study of U.S. adults with chronic illness. *Mental Health, Religion & Culture*. Advance online publication. https://doi.org/10.1080/13674676.2021.1948000

Fitzpatrick, S. J., Kerridge, I. H., Jordens, C. F. C., Zoloth, L., Tollefsen, C., Tsomo, K. L., Jensen, M. P., Sachedina, A., & Sarma, D. (2016). Religious perspectives on human suffering: Implications for medicine and bioethics. *Journal of Religion and Health, 55*(1), 159–173. https://doi.org/10.1007/s10943-015-0014-9

Govender, K., Cowden, R. G., Nyamaruze, P., Armstrong, R. M., & Hatane, L. (2020). Beyond the disease: Contextualized implications of the COVID-19 pandemic for children and young people living in Eastern and Southern Africa. *Frontiers in Public Health, 8*, 504. https://doi.org/10.3389/fpubh.2020.00504

Hamid, W., & Jahangir, M. S. (2020). Dying, death and mourning amid COVID-19 pandemic in Kashmir: A qualitative study. *OMEGA—Journal of Death and Dying*, 0030222820953708. https://doi.org/10.1177/0030222820953708

Hidalgo, M. C., & Hernández, B. (2001). Place attachment: Conceptual and empirical questions. *Journal of Environmental Psychology, 21*(3), 273–281. https://doi.org/10.1006/jevp.2001.0221

John Paul, I. I. (1984). *Apostolic letter: Salvifici doloris*. Holy See Press Office. Retrieved from http://www.vatican.va/content/john-paul-ii/en/apost_letters/1984/documents/hf_jp-ii_apl_11021984_salvifici-doloris.html

Jorgensen, B. S., & Stedman, R. C. (2001). Sense of place as an attitude: Lakeshore owners attitudes toward their properties. *Journal of Environmental Psychology, 21*(3), 233–248. https://doi.org/10.1006/jevp.2001.0226

Korpela, K. M. (2012). Place attachment. In S. D. Clayton (Ed.), *The Oxford handbook of environmental and conservation psychology* (pp. 148–163). Oxford University Press. https://doi.org/10.1093/oxfordhb/9780199733026.013.0009

Lewicka, M. (2011). Place attachment: How far have we come in the last 40 years? *Journal of Environmental Psychology, 31*(3), 207–230. https://doi.org/10.1016/j.jenvp.2010.10.001

Li, T. E., & Chan, E. T. H. (2018). Connotations of ancestral home: An exploration of place attachment by multiple generations of Chinese diaspora. *Population, Space and Place, 24*(8), e2147. https://doi.org/10.1002/psp.2147

Marroquín, B., Vine, V., & Morgan, R. (2020). Mental health during the COVID-19 pandemic: Effects of stay-at-home policies, social distancing behavior, and social resources. *Psychiatry Research, 293*, 113419. https://doi.org/10.1016/j.psychres.2020.113419

Mazumdar, S. & Mazumdar, S. (2004). Religion and place attachment: A study of sacred places. *Journal of Environmental Psychology, 24*(3), 385–397. https://doi.org/10.1016/j.jenvp.2004.08.005

Mobin-Uddin, A. (2018). An Islamic perspective: Suffering and meaning in cancer. *Clinical Journal of Oncology Nursing, 22*(5), 573–575. https://doi.org/10.1188/18.CJON.573-575

Pargament, K. I. (2001). *The psychology of religion and coping: Theory, research, practice*. Guilford Press.

Peng, J., Strijker, D., & Wu, Q. (2020). Place identity: How far have we come in exploring its meanings? *Frontiers in Psychology, 11*, 294. https://doi.org/10.3389/fpsyg.2020.00294

Ramkissoon, H. (2020). COVID-19 place confinement, pro-social, pro-environmental behaviors, and residents' wellbeing: A new conceptual framework. *Frontiers in Psychology, 11*, 2248. https://doi.org/10.3389/fpsyg.2020.02248

Scannell, L., Cox, R. S., Fletcher, S., & Heykoop, C. (2016). "That was the last time I saw my house": The importance of place attachment among children and youth in disaster contexts. *American Journal of Community Psychology, 58*(1–2), 158–173. https://doi.org/10.1002/ajcp.12069

Scannell, L., & Gifford, R. (2010). Defining place attachment: A tripartite organizing framework. *Journal of Environmental Psychology, 30*(1), 1–10. https://doi.org/10.1016/j.jenvp.2009.09.006

Scannell, L., & Gifford, R. (2016). Place attachment enhances psychological need satisfaction. *Environment and Behavior, 49*(4), 359–389. https://doi.org/10.1177/0013916516637648

Scannell, L., & Gifford, R. (2017). The experienced psychological benefits of place attachment. *Journal of Environmental Psychology, 51*, 256–269. https://doi.org/10.1016/j.jenvp.2017.04.001

Scannell, L., Williams, E., Gifford, R., & Sarich, C. (2021). Parallels between interpersonal and place attachment: An update. In L. C. Manzo & P. Devine-Wright (Eds.), *Place attachment: Advances in theory, methods, and applications* (2nd ed., pp. 45–60). Routledge.

Schopenhauer, A. (1909). *The world as will and idea* (Vol. 3, 6th ed.). (R. B. Haldane & J. Kemp, Trans.). Kegan Paul, Trench, Trübner & Co.

Sime, J. D. (1986). Creating places or designing spaces? *Journal of Environmental Psychology, 6*(1), 49–63. https://doi.org/10.1016/S0272-4944(86)80034-2

Tate, T., & Pearlman, R. (2019). What we mean when we talk about suffering–and why Eric Cassell should not have the last word. *Perspectives in Biology and Medicine, 62*(1), 95–110. https://doi.org/10.1353/pbm.2019.0005

Teasdale, J. D., & Chaskalson, M. (2011). How does mindfulness transform suffering? I: The nature and origins of dukkha. *Contemporary Buddhism, 12*(1), 89–102. https://doi.org/10.1080/14639947.2011.564824

Van Gordon, W., Shonin, E., Griffiths, M. D., & Singh, N. N. (2015). Mindfulness and the four noble truths. In E. Shonin, W. Van Gordon, & N. N. Singh (Eds.), *Buddhist foundations of mindfulness* (pp. 9–27). Springer. https://doi.org/10.1007/978-3-319-18591-0_2

van Tilburg, T. G., Steinmetz, S., Stolte, E., van der Roest, H., & de Vries, D. H. (2020). Loneliness and mental health during the COVID-19 pandemic: A study among Dutch older adults. *The Journals of Gerontology: Series B*, gbaa111. https://doi.org/10.1093/geronb/gbaa111

VanderWeele, T. J. (2019). Suffering and response: Directions in empirical research. *Social Science & Medicine, 224*, 58–66. https://doi.org/10.1016/j.socscimed.2019.01.041

VanderWeele, T. J. (2020). Love of neighbor during a pandemic: Navigating the competing goods of religious gatherings and physical health. *Journal of Religion and Health, 59*, 2196–2202. https://doi.org/10.1007/s10943-020-01031-6

Walsh, R. (1995). The problem of suffering: Existential and transpersonal perspectives. *The Humanistic Psychologist, 23*(3), 345–357. https://doi.org/10.1080/08873267.1995.9986835

Whitman, S. M. (2007). Pain and suffering as viewed by the Hindu religion. *The Journal of Pain, 8*(8), 607–613. https://doi.org/10.1016/j.jpain.2007.02.430

World Health Organization. (2021, March 23). *WHO coronavirus disease (COVID-19) dashboard*. Retrieved from https://covid19.who.int/

Chapter 5
Protest, Despair, and Detachment: Reparative Responses to Place Attachment Disruptions During a Pandemic

Victor Counted, Richard G. Cowden, and Haywantee Ramkissoon

Contents

Background on Place Attachment Disruption	55
Place Attachment Disruption During the COVID-19 Pandemic	57
Disrupted Place Attachment at Multiple Spatial Domains During a Pandemic	58
Reparative Responses to Place Attachment Disruption During a Pandemic	60
Protest	60
Despair	63
Detachment	64
Conclusion	66
References	66

In Chapter 1, we introduced place as a relational object of attachment. This conceptualization of place allows us to consider what happens when a global pandemic threatens the bonds that people have with places of significance. It also provides a framework for understanding how separation from a place of significance can lead to a reparative process in which people either rebuild their sense of connection to the place of attachment that has been disrupted or replace that attachment bond with an alternative attachment object. Using the framework offered by Counted et al. (2021), this chapter will explore the three theorized response phases—protest, despair, and detachment—that follow place attachment disruption.

Background on Place Attachment Disruption

Separation from a place of attachment may trigger separation distress (Counted, 2018; Counted & Zock, 2019). During the COVID-19 pandemic, separation distress may arise after being physically separated from a place that is part of our daily rounds or when our bond with a place has been threatened by pandemic-related public health measures. Hence, it is not necessary for a person to physically leave a place before they experience separation distress. For example, the safety precaution of remaining confined to one's home and not being able to access a place of significance could cause separation distress. We reason that any experience which challenges the norms of the inside–outside place dialectic may lead to some form of separation distress. When a person is separated from a place of attachment, reparative responses that culminate in maladaptive or adaptive outcomes may ensue. This phenomenon has been discussed in the attachment literature as *attachment disruption* (Kobak et al., 2016).

In one of the first studies on attachment, Bowlby et al. (1952) observed the responses of a 2-year-old girl, Laura, during an 8-day period when she was separated from her mother to have a minor operation. Throughout the time she was separated from her mother, Laura displayed separation anxiety and fretting as she monitored whether her mother would return and respond to her distress. Based on their observations, Bowlby et al. (1952) classified Laura's vicarious responses to being separated from her mother as phases of protest, despair, and detachment, which were the reparative responses employed by the child to "monitor danger in the environment, explore new learning opportunities, and enjoy social exchanges" when she was separated from her mother (Kobak et al., 2016, p. 27).

Before introducing, describing, and applying the three attachment disruption response phases to place attachment, it is important to first highlight a few overarching conceptual considerations. We theorize that all three phases associated with attachment disruption intersect cognitive, affective, and behavioral aspects of human experience. However, the salience of each aspect may vary based on the phenomenological attachment disruption experience of an individual within each phase. For example, both protest and despair phases involve some form of behavioral expression, but the type, extent, and intensity of negative affect experienced in each phase will differ across people. Although behavioral expressions will often provide insight into the dominant reparative phase that a person is processing, we suggest that these three phases are primarily distinguishable by the underlying cognitive-affective experience of a person within each phase. For example, behavioral expressions corresponding to both protest and despair phases may be similar, but the cognitive and affective underpinnings of the behavior will be quite distinct. It may not be possible to distinguish between the phases by focusing exclusively on behavior because "transitions" from one phase to another are likely to be fluid and could be nonlinear.

The *protest* phase that follows attachment disruption begins when one's object of attachment is no longer available to satisfy the bond of attachment, which can evoke "protest-like" behaviors that demonstrate dissatisfaction with the separation experience and the need to reconnect with the object. The *despair* phase occurs when the attached individual fears that their connection with the object of attachment has been lost and their hope of re-establishing that connection diminishes. This can be a very fragile phase, particularly for people with insecure working models of attachment who may experience a period of *deep mourning* that is characterized by intense anguish (Kobak et al., 2016). However, the *detachment* phase presents an opportunity for the person to explore other experiences and relationships that may transcend the lost attachment, marking the final stage of the reparative process. In the case of

Laura, she began turning to nurses and other people for support while she was separated from her maternal caregiver. Laura's incipient positive attitude toward other people and experiences was her way of coping with the difficulty of being separated from her mother.

Although Bowlby et al.'s (1952) work revealed how children tend to cope with the experience of being separated from a caregiver attachment figure, the observations reported in that research have not yet been extended to adult attachment experiences. We argue that insights gained from the work of Bowlby and colleagues apply to place attachment disruption experiences, including those that have transpired during the COVID-19 pandemic. Hence, adults may attempt to compensate for what has been lost during an experience of pandemic-related attachment disruption by exploring new relationships and alternative experiences (Counted et al., 2021). In this chapter, we explore the phases of protest, despair, and detachment in relation to place attachment disruptions that have taken place during the COVID-19 pandemic. In doing so, we suggest that separation distress which accompanies attachment disruption applies not only to being separated from a *human* attachment object but may also occur when a person is separated from a place of attachment.

Place Attachment Disruption During the COVID-19 Pandemic

Bowlby et al.'s (1952) seminal study is a valuable foundation from which to explore expressions of protest, despair, and detachment as signals of the emotional distress that accompanies separation from a place of attachment. The protest phase that follows place attachment disruption starts the moment a person feels their connection with a place of significance (e.g., places of worship, workplaces, university campuses) is dissipating. Within the context of the COVID-19 pandemic, phases of protest have been precipitated by public health measures that restricted people from engaging in non-essential activities outside of their homes. Behavioral responses in the protest phase may signify attempts by people to "hold onto" the experiences they are used to having in a particular place. The despair phase may have some overlap with the protest phase, such as when people voice their dissatisfaction with strategies implemented to limit or control the spread of SARS-CoV-2 (e.g., wearing of face masks). In some cases, the despair phase may involve a period of intense grief (Bowlby, 1969) over the experience of being separated from a place of attachment during the COVID-19 pandemic. Heinicke and Westheimer (1966) observed hostile behavioral patterns directed toward other people or objects in the despair phase. People who interpret their inability to access places of attachment as a catastrophe may engage in despair behaviors that resonate with the desperation or hopelessness they feel about not being able to regain access to a place of attachment that has been disrupted by the public health crisis. In the detachment phase, people begin to re-imagine a place of attachment or find new objects (e.g., virtual spaces, God) as alternative forms of attachment.

Separation from a place of attachment can occur through human-made and natural events (Counted, 2021). Human-made origins of place attachment disruption (e.g., civil conflict, economic crises, human rights violations) are usually caused by a combination of factors, such as economic inequality, injustice, marginalization, ethnic prejudice, and religious intolerance. Place attachment disruption can also apply to locals who perceive their sense of attachment to their home countries or neighborhoods affected by immigration and globalization forces. Place attachment disruptions also emanate from natural events, such as public health crises, weather-related disasters (e.g., hurricanes), environmental pollution, and climate change. These kinds of natural events are more common in countries and regions where extreme forces of nature threaten places of attachment by altering the natural environment.

The COVID-19 pandemic represents an event that is both natural and human-made. It is a natural event because current evidence indicates that SARS-CoV-2 had its origin in bats (Hayes, 2020). However, the COVID-19 pandemic is also a human-made event because SARS-CoV-2 has spread throughout the world due to a lack of transparency among countries and uncoordinated containment efforts. Many countries that have experienced a high burden of COVID-19 did not act swiftly enough to contain the transmission of SARS-CoV-2 early on. Delayed decisions by governments to close state and international borders, defiant behavior of people who disregarded stay-at-home orders, and propagation of conspiracy theories by influential people, groups, and communities all contributed to a high burden of disease in various parts of the world (Counted et al., 2021; Douglas, 2021). Although these are just a few factors that advanced the rapid, global spread of SARS-CoV-2, they highlight some of the reasons that the COVID-19 pandemic and its catastrophic consequences have been lingering for more than a year. Owing to both natural and human-made contributing factors, the public health crisis has disrupted many different bonds that people share with places that were formerly part of their daily lives.

Disrupted Place Attachment at Multiple Spatial Domains During a Pandemic

Place attachment occurs in three main spatial domains that intersect individual, social, cultural, and geographical aspects. These have been conceptualized as the place, person, and process domains (Scannell & Gifford, 2010). The place domain refers to a person's connection with the natural environment and geographical attributes of a place, such as the architecture of a city or buildings that make a city unique. Similar types of attachment can be formed with the beauty of nature and objects within the physical environment that are attractive or appealing to people. Research has found that the place domain is associated with excitement, boredom, fear, and relaxation (Fornara et al., 2010).

The person domain of place attachment refers to the experiences, interactions, lifeforms, milestones, and activities that are experienced in a particular place. These are things that people do in a place that make it special and unique, such as participating in religious rituals, growing up in a particular city or region, or moving to a specific place for a revered employment opportunity. These experiences and memories are often a central part of the thread that stitches together our bonds with places. By marking out spaces of meaning and experiences that help bring about place attachment, the person domain of place attachment reveals how places hold lifeworlds together spatially.

The process domain captures the conscious and unconscious psychological processes concerning the places that are an important part of a person's life. This aspect of place is intertwined with the person domain because experiences and memories in a place can "make a person." According to Proshansky et al. (1983), our place identity and understanding of who we are "extends with no less importance to objects and things and the very spaces and places in which they are found" (p. 57). Therefore, experiences and memories in a place can shape who we become and how we actively engage with place in general. The process domain is the cognitive component that contributes to identity development and continuity once an attachment has been established with a place. For example, a person from London may continue to have a strong connection to the city because of its urban culture, even if they no longer spend time in the city. Hence, people can hold onto and maintain a connection with a place that was once a large part of their lives.

The COVID-19 pandemic has had a substantial impact on the three domains of place attachment. Governments around the world enforced international travel restrictions and strict social distancing measures to limit the spread of SARS-CoV-2 (Govender et al., 2020). Many people who frequently traveled to certain places (e.g., workplaces, holiday destinations) before the public health crisis were no longer able to do so because access to public spaces was restricted. Popular local and international tourist destinations all over the world were no longer accessible (Ramkissoon, 2020). Businesses, schools, and other institutions (e.g., churches) were forced to close or continue operations remotely. By limiting our access to *physical* locations, these kinds of restrictions can lead to place attachment disruption within the place domain (Counted et al., 2021).

The public health crisis has disrupted the person domain of place attachment because it has changed how we experience places of significance. For example, many in-person events and cultural experiences (e.g., festivals, church gatherings) were canceled, postponed, or shifted to online formats. Public health measures included limits on non-essential travel and public social gatherings, which have made it difficult for people to individually and collectively experience places in the ways they did before the COVID-19 pandemic. Hence, the public health crisis has made it challenging for people to truly connect with the experiences, cultural lifeforms, and memories that are tethered to their places of attachment.

The COVID-19 pandemic has also impacted the process domain because people often have place identities rooted in places that are habitually part of their lives (Counted et al., 2021). A person's place identity is fluid and tends to evolve gradually, which means that pandemic-related place attachment disruption within the process domain may be less devastating compared to the place and person domains. However, place identity might take on new forms of meaning as people explore alternative avenues to maintain their connections with places of significance. People are using virtual mediums to find new ways of learning about themselves outside of physical places that were formerly a large part of their lives (Bowles, 2020). Technologically assisted changes to place identity have been made possible by the duration of the lockdowns that left many people largely confined to their homes for an extended period of time. Although transforming place identity by shedding aspects of the self that were rooted in a particular place may be necessary for self-continuity and can be an adaptive response that supports coping during a period of loss (Sadeh & Karniol, 2012), some people may struggle with identity changes and self-disembodiment as they try to hold onto the comfort of their existing place-based identity (Counted et al., 2021).

Reparative Responses to Place Attachment Disruption During a Pandemic

Place attachment disruptions within the context of the COVID-19 pandemic have intersected the place, person, and process domains of place attachment. Figure 5.1 provides a visual depiction of how place attachment disruption experiences during the public health crisis may have elicited a multifaceted reparative process characterized by phases of protest, despair, and detachment. We briefly introduce and discuss some of the ways that each of these three phases may have unfolded in the aftermath of pandemic-related place attachment disruption experiences.

Protest

According to Kobak et al. (2016), the protest phase begins when the object of attachment "switches off" communication with the care seeker. The protest phase signals that the person is in a state of separation distress. For infants, protest can be exhibited through behavior such as crying loudly to get the attention of the caregiver or clinging to the caregiver to prevent separation (Bowlby et al., 1952; Kobak et al., 2016). Thus, protest behaviors are attention-seeking efforts that children engage in to signal separation distress. For adults who have a bond with a particular place, the protest phase that accompanies their experience of place attachment disruption will likely involve an attention-seeking response to the distress of being separated from or unable to access a place of significance. Even though a person may be experiencing separation distress and displaying defiant emotional responses (e.g., anger)

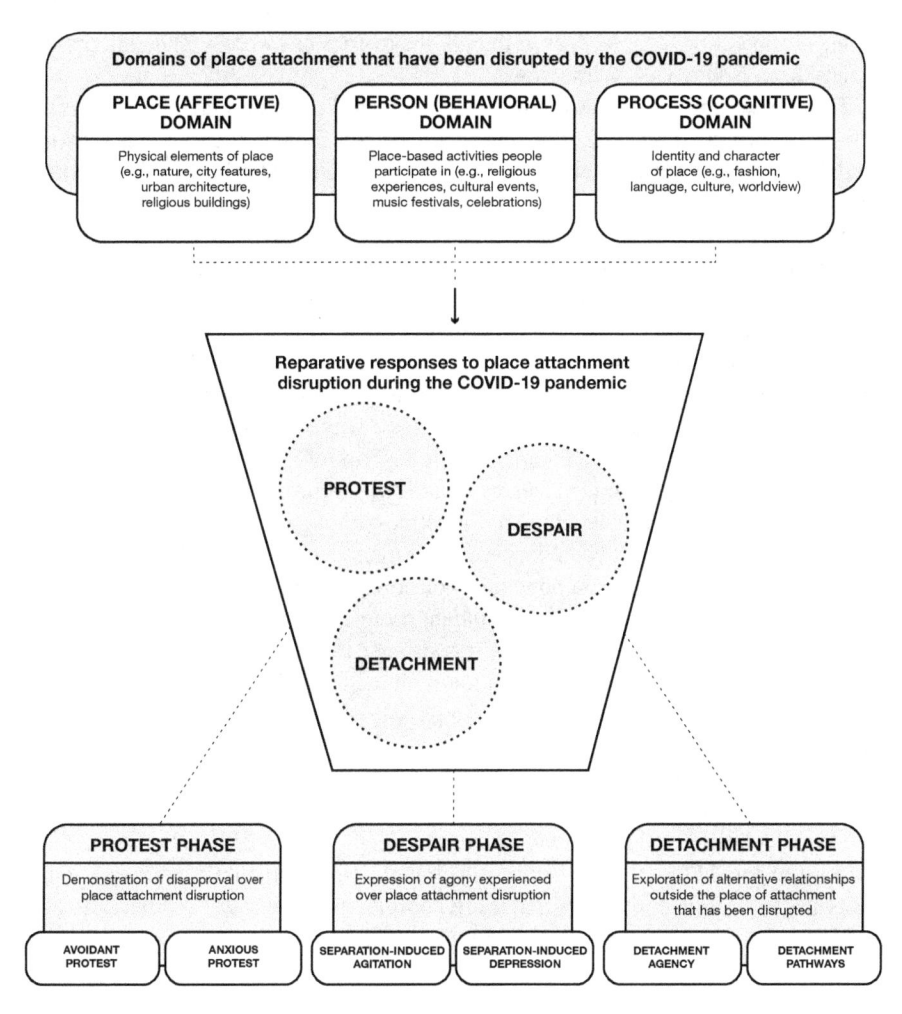

Fig. 5.1 Framework of reparative responses to place attachment disruption during the COVID-19 pandemic

during this phase, they may still be hopeful about reconnecting with the object of attachment.

Place attachment disruption caused by the COVID-19 pandemic may elicit a behavioral demonstration of protest. For example, some people might ignore, disregard, or intentionally flout pandemic-related public health measures to express their separation distress and "protest" their place attachment disruption. Behavioral responses within the protest phase reflect the attempts of people to conserve or re-establish their attachment bonds with places that were a significant part of their lives before the COVID-19 pandemic. The intention behind these kinds of behaviors is to get the attention of those who implemented stringent measures that inhibit the flow of one's connection to a place, even though the restrictions were intended to protect society from SARS-CoV-2 infection.

The protest phase that follows place attachment disruption may be shaped by a person's working model of attachment. In the attachment literature, a working model is a mental representation of the world, oneself, and others. This cognitive framework of representation can determine whether a person responds to separation distress insecurely or in a mature, secure fashion. Drawing on research involving human attachment figures (Bartholomew & Shaver, 1998; Davis et al., 2003; Finzi et al., 2001), it is possible that insecurely attached individuals with an anxious working model will have a greater proclivity to respond to place attachment disruptions with protest, even when the threat to their attachment bond is relatively benign. Similarly, people characterized by an insecure-avoidant attachment style may be more inclined to avoid a place of attachment as a way of dealing with the threat of place attachment disruption. Given our prior description of the attachment working model, we propose that anxious and avoidant forms of protest may arise in response to pandemic-related place attachment disruptions among people who are insecurely attached. Although protest behaviors may take many forms, in this chapter we focus on a few of the more common potential protest responses.

As described in Counted (2021), avoidant protest responses can include passive-aggressiveness (e.g., concealed or covert resistance to public safety regulations) and rumination (e.g., unhealthy preoccupation with the loss of place resources). Within the context of the COVID-19 pandemic, a passive-aggressive form of avoidant protest can trigger an "unspoken" resistance toward public health measures (e.g., unwillingness to wear a mask in public). Rumination is a stressful form of avoidant protest that involves replaying the causes, situational factors, or consequences of pandemic-related place attachment disruption (e.g., existential questions about the purpose of the COVID-19 pandemic). Although it is often subtle, rumination can become the genesis of a bigger and more complex psychological problem. As two forms of avoidant protest, passive-aggressiveness and rumination are defense mechanisms that people with insecure-avoidant attachment styles may rely on to avoid confronting the reality of their pandemic-related place attachment disruption experience.

The distress that a person experiences in response to place attachment disruption can also be expressed through a variety of anxious responses, such as clingy or needy behaviors. For example, some individuals may attempt to visit a place that holds significant value to them even if the location is situated in a COVID-19 hotspot where the risk of SARS-CoV-2 infection is particularly high. This might explain why some people disregarded stay-at-home orders and non-essential travel restrictions during the COVID-19 pandemic. Although the primary objective of an anxious form of protest would be to maintain a sense of connection with a place of attachment, it could cause further disruption to a pre-existing relationship with a place when the protest behavior is met with an escalation of public health measures that more strictly enforce limits on access to a place.

Both avoidant and anxious forms of protest can be traced to the inner working models of attachment. Regardless of how each form of protest manifests at cognitive, affective, and behavioral levels, avoidant and anxious protest responses are defensive mechanisms that people rely on to cope with their experiences of place attachment disruption. Although these two protest responses serve adaptive functions of attempting to maintain a person's bond with a place of attachment, they could also lead to additional stress that activates the phase of despair.

Despair

The despair phase begins when a person loses all hope of maintaining their connection with a place of attachment. Although this phase of the reparative process will more commonly involve the painful kinds of emotions that accompany experiences of loss (e.g., sadness), hostile behaviors may be observed (Heinicke & Westheimer, 1966). Similar to how a child might throw aside objects that remind them of the caregiver from whom they have been separated, adult responses in the despair phase may include antagonistic or violent behaviors toward people or objects that remind a person of the attachment relationship they have lost (Counted, 2021). According to attachment literature, insecurely attached individuals will be at increased risk of responding to attachment disruption with despair because of their emotional vulnerability (Bartholomew & Shaver, 1998; Kobak et al., 2016). For example, anxiously attached individuals may become inconsolable in response to having their connection with a place severed, which could spiral into a relentless state of misery. In contrast, avoidantly attached individuals may bypass the despair phase by attempting to swiftly "let go" of a place attachment bond without first going through the process of grieving the attachment relationship that has been lost.

In the despair phase, people may progress from initial signs of separation-induced agitation to a state of separation-induced depression (Counted, 2021). Separation-induced agitation is triggered by the shock of realizing that one's relationship with a specific place of attachment may not be salvageable (Kobak & Bosmans, 2019; Kobak et al., 2016). It arises from the agony that is experienced when mourning a loss of attachment (Heinicke & Westheimer, 1966). In response, people adopt agitated behaviors to soothe the emotional pain that follows the realization that one's bond with an attachment object has been permanently severed. Separation-induced agitation may be expressed as distress vocalizations or restless kinds of behaviors (e.g., impulsivity). On the other hand, separation-induced depression refers to experiences of emptiness, hopelessness, or grief over the perceived or actual permanent separation from an object of attachment (Bowlby et al., 1952; Heinicke & Westheimer, 1966). The intensity of separation-induced depression can be unbearable (Kobak et al., 2016), with some people at risk of entering a dangerous state of mind because they are unable to "separate" themselves from the profound, persistent, and all-consuming state of sorrow. We discuss how these two aspects of the despair phase might be experienced in response to place attachment disruption that occurs within the context of the COVID-19 pandemic.

In the despair phase, separation-induced agitation may involve distress vocalizations that reflect a person's displeasure with anything that they feel has cost them their place attachment bond (Counted, 2021). Some people may publicly voice their anguish over how community mitigation strategies designed to control transmission of SARS-CoV-2 have upended their attachment to place. Others may rebuke government authorities or adamantly express their loss of confidence in their governments for enacting public health measures that restrain their mobility and limit social gatherings in public spaces. Although distress vocalizations will be the more common kinds of separation-induced agitation behaviors exhibited by people who feel they are no longer able to stay connected to a place of attachment during the COVID-19 pandemic, more radical forms of separation-induced agitation are also possible. For example, a person may display separation-induced agitation by using social media platforms (e.g., Twitter, Facebook) to deliberately spread misinformation about the public health crisis or incite violence.

Separation-induced depression in the despair phase that follows pandemic-related place attachment disruption will usually entail feelings of sadness and a sense of hopelessness over losing a place of attachment (Counted, 2021). Some people may show signs that closely reflect their underlying state of separation-induced depression, such as avoidance of social interactions, apathy, or lethargy. In more extreme cases, separation-induced depression can be overwhelming and may culminate in hostility toward other people (e.g., family members) or self-harming behaviors. Those kinds of behaviors reflect attempts by people to transfer their negative emotions or "escape" the deep state of misery caused by pandemic-related place attachment disruption. If people who have experienced place attachment disruption during the COVID-19 pandemic are able to effectively cope with and successfully work through separation-induced depression, they may be more likely to build alternative forms of attachment bonds in the detachment phase.

Detachment

Transcending place attachment disruptions caused by the COVID-19 pandemic may require engaging in detachment behavior (Counted et al., 2021), which is when the attached person starts to explore other attachment objects (Kobak et al., 2016). During this phase, the individual is able to mentally disconnect from the place of attachment and find new ways of achieving attachment goals outside of the place attachment bond that may have been lost, compromised, or can no longer be repaired or restored. Even though the detachment phase is what enables people to ultimately transcend their place attachment disruption experience, it may be a complicated and challenging phase to work through. Similar to the protest and despair phases, a person's inner working model of attachment will shape how they progress through the detachment phase (Counted, 2021; Counted et al., 2021). For example, people with insecure working models of attachment may find it highly stressful to explore new, prospective forms of relationships, which could increase their risk of returning to the despair phase if their initial attempts at building new attachment bonds are not successful. Hence, it is important to consider the different ways in which people may advance through the detachment phase toward successful resolution of a place attachment disruption experience.

The detachment phase of pandemic-related place attachment disruption may take different forms. Here, we focus on hope as a means of detaching from a place of attachment that may be out of a person's reach because of how the COVID-19 pandemic has limited access to places within the environment. According to Snyder's (2000, 2002) goal-focused theory, hope requires the agency to execute desired goals (i.e., willpower) and the ability to generate pathways toward achieving those goals (i.e., waypower). Agency is an intrinsic aspect of hope that has to do with having the self-efficacy to achieve desired goals, whereas the pathways component is more extrinsic because one has to bring hopeful expectations to reality by identifying resources and strategies to achieve desired goals (Counted et al., 2020). Both the agency and pathway aspects of hope are necessary for successfully overcoming place attachment disruption, as a person needs hopeful thinking and action to effectively explore new, unfamiliar, and corrective relationships to compensate for the disrupted bond with a particular place.

Snyder's (2000, 2002) goal-focused theory of hope provides a framework for understanding detachment as an adaptive response that starts with hope. To draw on hope as a means of detaching from a place that no longer aligns with our attachment goals, one must find a new corrective detachment object, have the self-agency to attain and execute desired detachment goals, and be able to access pathways that allow them to transcend their place attachment disruption experience. Detachment starts with exploring new objects of attachment, but it requires willpower to attain and sustain a meaningful connection with a new object of attachment that supports well-being.

In response to place attachment disruption during the COVID-19 pandemic, people may be able to amass the willpower needed to detach from places that were a significant part of their lives (e.g., schools, workplaces, places of worship). For example, some people may be able to disconnect mentally and emotionally from a place that no longer serves their needs by turning to virtual spaces, which afford a greater sense of personal control over interactions with "places" compared to many physical places that have been rendered inaccessible during the COVID-19 pandemic. However, others may require resources (e.g., social support) to generate pathways that facilitate detachment from a place of attachment and provide opportunities for alternative forms of attachment bonds to develop (e.g., relationship with God). By accessing pathways and harnessing personal agency to detach from a place of attachment that has been disrupted by the COVID-19 pandemic, new relationship experiences could ignite, renew, or strengthen a person's sense of purpose and meaning in life.

Conclusion

Place attachment disruption can elicit a multiphased reparative process involving affective, cognitive, and behavioral constituents. Drawing on Counted et al.'s (2021) framework of place attachment disruption, this chapter discussed protest, despair, and detachment as phases that are experienced after a place attachment disruption that has transpired during the COVID-19 pandemic. Each of these phases is considered a necessary part of the process of working through a place attachment disruption experience, which in many cases will culminate in the formation of new attachment bonds. However, place attachment disruption is a phenomenological experience that is influenced by a range of interfacing components, such as individual (e.g., inner workings of a person's attachment behavioral system), environmental (e.g., the type of place that a person is separated from), and institutional factors (e.g., stringency of public health measures imposed by governments). The impact of the COVID-19 pandemic on humanity has been devastating, but it has also provided us with an opportunity to better understand place attachment disruption experiences and the dynamic ways in which responses to place attachment disruption may manifest. There is much potential for the lessons we have learned about experiences of place attachment disruption during the current public health crisis to inform public health initiatives or psychotherapeutic programs that can be used to support people both during and after the COVID-19 pandemic.

References

Bartholomew, K., & Shaver, P. R. (1998). Methods of assessing adult attachment: Do they converge? In J. A. Simpson & W. S. Rholes (Eds.), *Attachment theory and close relationships* (pp. 25–45). Guilford Press.

Bowlby, J. (1969). *Attachment and loss: Attachment* (Vol. 1). Basic Books.

Bowlby, J., Robertson, J., & Rosenbluth, D. (1952). A two-year-old goes to hospital. *The Psychoanalytic Study of the Child, 7*(1), 82–94. https://doi.org/10.1080/00797308.1952.11823154

Bowles, T. (2020, July 20). *Our changing identities under COVID-19*. Pursuit. Retrieved from https://pursuit.unimelb.edu.au/articles/our-changing-identities-under-covid-19

Counted, V. (2018). The Circle of Place Spirituality (CoPS): Towards an attachment and exploration motivational systems approach in the psychology of religion. In A. Village & R. W. Hood (Eds.), *Research in the social scientific study of religion* (Vol. 29, pp. 145–174). Brill. https://doi.org/10.1163/9789004382640_009

Counted, V. (2021). *The roots of radicalization: Disrupted attachment systems and displacement*. Lexington Books.

Counted, V., Neff, M. A., Captari, L. E., & Cowden, R. G. (2021). Transcending place attachment disruptions during a public health crisis: Spiritual struggles, resilience, and transformation. *Journal of Psychology and Christianity, 39*(4), 276–286.

Counted, V., Pargament, K. I., Bechara, A. O., Joynt, S., & Cowden, R. G. (2020). Hope and well-being in vulnerable contexts during the COVID-19 pandemic: Does religious coping matter? *The Journal of Positive Psychology*. Advance online publication. https://doi.org/10.1080/17439760.2020.1832247

Counted, V., & Zock, H. T. (2019). Place spirituality: An attachment perspective. *Archive for the Psychology of Religion, 41*(1), 12–25. https://doi.org/10.1177/0084672419833448

Davis, D., Shaver, P. R., & Vernon, M. L. (2003). Physical, emotional, and behavioral reactions to breaking up: The roles of gender, age, emotional involvement, and attachment style. *Personality and Social Psychology Bulletin, 29*(7), 871–884. https://doi.org/10.1177/0146167203029007006

Douglas, K. M. (2021). COVID-19 conspiracy theories. *Group Processes & Intergroup Relations, 24*(2), 270–275. https://doi.org/10.1177/1368430220982068

Finzi, R., Ram, A., Har-Even, D., Shnit, D., & Weizman, A. (2001). Attachment styles and aggression in physically abused and neglected children. *Journal of Youth and Adolescence, 30*(6), 769–786. https://doi.org/10.1023/A:1012237813771

Fornara, F., Bonaiuto, M., & Bonnes, M. (2010). Cross-validation of abbreviated perceived residential environment quality (PREQ) and neighborhood attachment (NA) indicators. *Environment and Behavior, 42*(2), 171–196. https://doi.org/10.1177/0013916508330998

Govender, K., Cowden, R. G., Nyamaruze, P., Armstrong, R. M., & Hatane, L. (2020). Beyond the disease: Contextualized implications of the COVID-19 pandemic for children and young people living in Eastern and Southern Africa. *Frontiers in Public Health, 8*, 504. https://doi.org/10.3389/fpubh.2020.00504

Hayes, P. (2020, July 13). *Here's how scientists know the coronavirus came from bats and wasn't made in a lab*. The Conversation. Retrieved from https://theconversation.com/heres-how-scientists-know-the-coronavirus-came-from-bats-and-wasnt-made-in-a-lab-141850

Heinicke, C. M., & Westheimer, I. (1966). *Brief separations*. International University Press.

Kobak, R., & Bosmans, G. (2019). Attachment and psychopathology: A dynamic model of the insecure cycle. *Current Opinion in Psychology, 25*, 76–80. https://doi.org/10.1016/j.copsyc.2018.02.018

Kobak, R., Zajac, K., & Madsen, S. D. (2016). Attachment disruptions, reparative processes, and psychopathology. In J. Cassidy & P. R. Shaver (Eds.), *Handbook of attachment: Theory, research, and clinical applications* (3rd ed., pp. 25–39). Guilford Press.

Proshansky, H. M., Fabian, A. K., & Kaminoff, R. (1983). Place-identity: Physical world socialization of the self. *Journal of Environmental Psychology, 3*(1), 57–83. https://doi.org/10.1016/S0272-4944(83)80021-8

Ramkissoon, H. (2020). Perceived social impacts of tourism and quality-of-life: A new conceptual model. *Journal of Sustainable Tourism.* Advance online publication. https://doi.org/10.1080/09669582.2020.1858091

Sadeh, N., & Karniol, R. (2012). The sense of self-continuity as a resource in adaptive coping with job loss. *Journal of Vocational Behavior, 80*(1), 93–99. https://doi.org/10.1016/j.jvb.2011.04.009

Scannell, L., & Gifford, R. (2010). Defining place attachment: A tripartite organizing framework. *Journal of Environmental Psychology, 30*(1), 1–10. https://doi.org/10.1016/j.jenvp.2009.09.006

Snyder, C. R. (2000). The past and possible futures of hope. *Journal of Social and Clinical Psychology, 19*(1), 11–28. https://doi.org/10.1521/jscp.2000.19.1.11

Snyder, C. R. (2002). Hope theory: Rainbows in the mind. *Psychological Inquiry, 13*(4), 249–275. https://doi.org/10.1207/S15327965PLI1304_01

Part II
Adjusting to Place Attachment Disruption During and After a Pandemic

Chapter 6
Adapting to Place Attachment Disruption During a Pandemic: From Resource Loss to Resilience

Richard G. Cowden, Victor Counted, and Haywantee Ramkissoon

Contents

Psychological Distress of Place Attachment Disruption.	72
Rebounding from Resource Loss.	73
Mobilizing Religious/Spiritual Resources.	74
Building Religious/Spiritual Resources for Resilience.	76
Conclusion.	77
References.	77

The COVID-19 pandemic instigated a remarkable range of stressors that have impacted people all around the world (Cowden, Rueger, et al., 2021). Those stressors have affected economic (e.g., financial security), interpersonal (e.g., social connectedness), physical (e.g., health), psychological (e.g., mental well-being), and religious/spiritual (e.g., in-person religious services) domains of human life (Blustein et al., 2020; Dein et al., 2020; O'Connor et al., 2020; Xiong et al., 2020; Zhang et al., 2020). Pandemic-related stressors constitute different forms of resource loss, due in large part to the widespread community mitigation strategies (e.g., stay-at-home orders, physical distancing requirements) that have been enacted in countries and territories around the world to prevent or limit transmission of SARS-CoV-2.

One form of pandemic-related resource loss that is primarily attributable to the implementation of public health control measures is place attachment disruption, which arises when people are separated from a place of significance (Scannell et al., 2021). Drawing on an integrated resource theory, this chapter explores place attachment disruption during the COVID-19 pandemic as a form of resource loss that evokes psychological distress. It discusses the potential for resource acquisition and facilitation to buffer the negative effects of pandemic-related place attachment disruption, including some emphasis on the role of religion/spirituality in building resources that could guard against future loss.

Psychological Distress of Place Attachment Disruption

According to the COR theory, humans are motivated to acquire, retain, and protect valued resources (Hobfoll, 1989, 2001). Resources include anything a person perceives as being useful for goal attainment (Halbesleben et al., 2014), but can broadly be classified into superordinate categories of condition (e.g., good physical health, stable employment), energy (e.g., knowledge, time), personal (e.g., hope, self-efficacy), and object (e.g., a house, places of worship) resources (Hobfoll et al., 2018). Places of attachment might principally be understood as object resources (see Chapter 3), but they are usually linked to other types of resources (e.g., comfort and security, sense of belonging, means of personal growth) that people rely on to support their well-being (Scannell & Gifford, 2017).

Environmental demands that threaten or result in actual loss of resources can lead to psychological distress (Hobfoll et al., 2018). COR theory offers several points about resources that are particularly relevant for understanding how psychological distress might emerge from pandemic-related place attachment disruption. First, resources exist within an ecological context that can either support or block resources from being built, nurtured, or sustained (Holmgreen et al., 2017). During the COVID-19 pandemic, resource availability has been undermined by community mitigation strategies that have formed part of public health efforts to control the spread of SARS-CoV-2 (see Chapter 4). As many of those public health control measures have inadvertently separated people from places of attachment (e.g., places of worship, schools, workplaces), people have been restricted in their ability to access resources that are tethered to places of significance (Counted et al., 2021). Second, resources are often interconnected (Hobfoll et al., 2016). Certain resources develop from common environmental conditions, and resources often coexist within "resource caravans" (Doane et al., 2012). Hence, loss of one resource may be reciprocally related to loss of other types of resources (Hobfoll & Schumm, 2009).

Place attachment disruption offers a poignant representation of the interrelatedness of resource loss, as it usually interferes with a variety of resources connected to a place of significance (Scannell et al., 2016). Several studies have found that people can feel overwhelmed by the extent of resource loss that may transpire when separated from a place of attachment (Boğaç, 2009; Brown & Perkins, 1992). For some people, the destabilizing effects of having numerous resources threatened by pandemic-related place attachment disruption could lead to psychological distress (see Chapter 4). Third, resource loss can be challenging for people to deal with because it diminishes the reservoir of resources that one might need to successfully cope with future demands (Hobfoll & Schumm, 2009). In contexts where ongoing community mitigation strategies have disrupted place attachments for prolonged periods of time, people may find it difficult to cope with new stressors that emerge while separated from places of attachment. When pandemic-related place attachment disruption leaves a person with insufficient resource reserves to meet the demands they face during the public health crisis, a spiral of loss and psychological distress may follow.

Rebounding from Resource Loss

The psychological distress that follows resource loss signals to the person that resources are needed to offset the net loss (Doane et al., 2012). People may attempt to recover from resource loss through direct resource replacement or resource substitution (Hobfoll, 2001). When resource loss that arises from pandemic-related place attachment disruption centers on the physical aspects of the place itself, a person might counteract the loss by striving to replace the place of attachment with an alternative place that is more accessible (e.g., an outdoor location whose access is not restricted by public health control measures). If the resource that has been affected is secondary to the experience of being separated from a place of attachment (e.g., social connectedness), an individual may try to recover the loss through other avenues (e.g., online communities).

Although there may be instances in which direct resource replacement is sufficient for offsetting the kinds of resources that have been lost through place attachment disruption, an indirect approach might be needed when direct replacement is not a feasible option. Resource substitution refers to the replacement of a lost resource with an alternative resource that has the potential to meet the environmental demands arising from loss or threat of loss (Halbesleben et al., 2014). Depending on the loss that is precipitated by pandemic-related place attachment disruption, substitution may involve leveraging any number of internal or external resources that could contribute to offsetting loss. For example, people who have been separated from a place of attachment during the COVID-19 pandemic may attempt to substitute the psychological benefits (e.g., restorative experience) that a place of attachment usually provides by turning to interpersonal (e.g., family) or transcendental (e.g., God) resources for support. In Chapter 5, we discuss the concept of detachment as one type of resource substitution process.

Research suggests that people often rely on personal or social resources to offset event-related losses (Hobfoll, 2001). Although they are not the only resource reserves that people make use of, personal and social resources provide a useful illustration of how different combinations of resources might shape adjustment to pandemic-related place attachment disruption. Personal and social resources are interrelated, may affect one another, and the availability of each can influence how people attempt to cope with resource loss (Hobfoll & Schumm, 2009). Those who have an abundance of personal resources are not only more likely to possess social resources that they can call upon to effectively cope with environmental demands, but social resources can also strengthen personal resources. When a more abundant combination of personal and social resources is available, people have greater flexibility to select and use resources that provide the best opportunity for offsetting loss. A person may initially respond to loss that accompanies pandemic-related place attachment disruption by investing personal resources. However, if the demand outweighs personal resource reserves, then relevant social resources could be engaged to reduce the net resource loss gap. When a loss necessitates that both personal and social resources be employed, richer reserves of each can limit resource depletion because resources that are allocated may be diffused across both resource domains. Those who offset loss that emanates from place attachment disruption by engaging a combination of personal and social resources might be able to preserve a more diverse set of resources for dealing with subsequent stressors (e.g., job loss) that could emerge within the course of the COVID-19 pandemic.

Resource mobilization is a necessary undertaking for offsetting loss. Yet available resources may not always be sufficient to counteract, compensate for, or overcome loss (Holmgreen et al., 2017). When that occurs, people may attempt to conserve resources by engaging in cognitive processes that modify the way they think about the situation (Hobfoll, 2001). For example, a person may shift their focus away from what has been lost toward what might be gained (i.e., positive reframing), re-evaluate the loss from the vantage point of another person (i.e., self-distancing), or envision how a future self might perceive the loss (i.e., temporal distancing). These kinds of reappraisal techniques serve a self-regulatory function and have been shown to reduce psychological distress (Ranney et al., 2017). However, cognitive reappraisal may only be useful to the extent that a particular loss is open to personal appraisal. Some people who have dealt with pandemic-related place attachment disruption might experience it as a microstressor that constitutes an opportunity for personal growth. For others, it could elicit a catastrophic state of extensive loss that has little redemptive value. Cognitive reappraisal may yield limited benefits for those in the latter category, particularly if reappraisal processes juxtapose basic assumptions that a person has about themselves and the environment (Hobfoll, 1989).

Mobilizing Religious/Spiritual Resources

History suggests that religious/spiritual resources gain salience in times of crisis (Counted et al., 2020; Dein et al., 2020). The COVID-19 pandemic constitutes such a crisis, the consequences of which might be exacerbated among those who are burdened with navigating the challenges of the pandemic without being able to access place-based resources that usually support their needs. When pervasive resource loss is met with few tangible opportunities for gains that might offset such losses, religion/spirituality may form a central part of the resources that a person relies on to cope with stress (Counted et al., 2021; Pargament, 1997). The circumstances that arise from place attachment disruption that occurs during the COVID-19 pandemic may prompt many people to draw on their relationship with the sacred for comfort, safety, and security, seek or re-establish a relationship with the sacred, or strengthen their commitment to religious/spiritual beliefs and practices. Religious/spiritual resources may not be sufficient in themselves to offset resource loss that arises from pandemic-related place attachment disruption, but investment in religious/spiritual resources could cultivate other resources that offer more direct benefits. For example, religious/spiritual practices (e.g., prayer) may augment personal resources (e.g., hope) by facilitating positive meaning-making (Fredrickson, 2002), which could then be used to buffer the impact of resource loss that is attributable to place attachment disruption.

Many adherents of religious/spiritual traditions accustomed to gathering in physical locations have had their attachments to places of worship disrupted during the COVID-19 pandemic (see Chapter 4). Restrictions on social gatherings have led to the suspension of in-person religious services and closure of places of worship, forcing faith-based communities to find alternative ways of supporting the spiritual life of parishioners. As part of that response, there has been an exponential increase in virtual-based opportunities (e.g., online services, guided study of scripture, prayer gatherings) for people to participate in religious/spiritual activities during the public health crisis (Dein et al., 2020; Pew Research Center, 2020). Even though religious/spiritual life may only be partially fulfilled through online options (VanderWeele, 2020), the rapid rise in opportunities for online religious/spiritual engagement has paradoxically presented people with many alternative means of developing and maintaining spiritual well-being. Those dealing with losses associated with being separated from a place of worship may benefit from resources gained through online-based religious/spiritual participation (e.g., a strengthened sense of coherence). For people who have experienced place attachment disruption in other ways during the COVID-19 pandemic, participation in online religious/spiritual activities may be a bridge to useful resources (e.g., social support) that could facilitate recovery from losses.

Gains in religious/spiritual resources may have special relevance to people facing pandemic-related place attachment disruption in contexts where social-structural disadvantages (e.g., poverty, gender inequality) limit the availability of material resources. Social-structural constraints can make it difficult for people to access and accrue resources (Cowden et al., 2020; Govender et al., 2020). Although individuals who lack resources are more susceptible to resource loss and its implications, resource gains within vulnerable contexts may have a powerful impact on building resource gain momentum and a person's capacity to offset loss (Hobfoll et al., 2018). By turning to the sacred in the aftermath of pandemic-related place attachment disruption, people living in contexts of social-structural disadvantage may gain access to unique sources of strength that activate gain cycles. For example, rekindling connection to the sacred through religious/spiritual practices (e.g., prayer, reading scripture) could nurture personal resources (e.g., hope) that contribute to rebuilding conditional resources (e.g., mental well-being) that have been negatively impacted by pandemic-related place attachment disruption. Thus, gain cycles precipitated by an accrual of religious/spiritual resources may yield important dividends for people living in contexts where social-structural disadvantages that existed before the COVID-19 pandemic could make it more challenging to offset loss that arises during the public health crisis. However, religious/spiritual resources should not be considered a panacea for every loss that accompanies place attachment disruption, and there may even be instances when religion/spirituality is not particularly beneficial (Cowden, Rueger, et al., 2021).

Much like any other coping mechanism, the notion that religious/spiritual resources can help with offsetting loss should be considered alongside the potential for religion/spirituality to undermine recovery from resource loss (Pargament & Lomax, 2013). Some people who are confronted with resource loss experience religious/spiritual struggles in the form of tensions, strains, and conflicts about sacred matters with the supernatural, within oneself, and with other people (Exline, 2013; Cowden, Pargament, et al., 2021). For example, a person who is separated from a sacred place of significance during the COVID-19 pandemic may have lost access to a central part of their religious/spiritual life (Counted et al., 2021). Such loss could evoke religious/spiritual struggles, such as divine struggles (e.g., feeling as though one has been punished or abandoned by the sacred) or ultimate meaning struggles (e.g., a sense of meaninglessness about one's life). Religious/spiritual struggles are stressful because they are disruptive to the orienting system that characterizes how a person typically perceives, makes sense of, and interacts with the world around them (Pargament, 2007; Pargament & Ano, 2006). This can make it more difficult for people to cope with resource loss that accompanies pandemic-related place attachment disruption. Religious/spiritual struggles may also have a negative impact on the availability of other resources (e.g., social support) that might otherwise facilitate positive adjustment (Pargament et al., 2006), which could further complicate the recovery process of those who have experienced place attachment disruption during the COVID-19 pandemic.

Building Religious/Spiritual Resources for Resilience

Even though stressful situations challenge resources and may result in resource loss, benefits may emerge from the process of dealing with difficult circumstances. When resource loss transpires, people become more motivated to accrue resources (Hobfoll, 2002). Resource gains not only support recuperation from current loss, but they can also offer protection from future loss (Doane et al., 2012). Pandemic-related place attachment disruption could catalyze a transformative process characterized by resource gains in previously undiscovered or underdeveloped areas. One way that such transformation could be achieved is through detachment (see Chapter 5), which involves developing or strengthening other forms of relationships that are outside the place of attachment that has been disrupted (Counted et al., 2021). Detachment may take different forms, such as reinforcing attachment to one's home or establishing new social bonds. With the public health crisis bringing concerns about human fragility and finitude into sharp focus (Cowden, Davis, et al., 2021), people who are confronted with pandemic-related place attachment disruption might be especially motivated to pursue the sacred as a form of detachment.

Relationship with the sacred often provides people with a sense of safety, comfort, and solutions to problems that corporeal resources may not be able to adequately address (Counted, 2018; Wong et al., 2018). Non-adherents of religious/spiritual traditions may seek connection with the sacred as a new source of external support for coping with pandemic-related place attachment disruption, whereas people of faith may reaffirm their relationship with the sacred to build on existing transcendental resources (Counted et al., 2021). Gains in religious/spiritual resources can protect against future loss because stressful life events often lead to the development of religious/spiritual resources that people bring with them to cope with hardships that occur over time (Manning, 2013; Shaw et al., 2005). People who accumulate religious/spiritual resources in the process of navigating pandemic-related place attachment disruption may be better equipped to handle subsequent stressors, including other experiences of place attachment disruption.

Conclusion

Separation from a place of attachment during the COVID-19 pandemic may constitute a disruptive form of loss that can have negative implications for well-being. A natural response is to employ resources to regain, replace, or otherwise compensate for such loss (Holmgreen et al., 2017). This chapter has explored some of the ways that people who have encountered pandemic-related place attachment disruption may attempt to recover from accompanying losses. Although a central purpose of resource mobilization is to offset current loss, resources that are gained through the process of dealing with stressful life events have the potential to support positive adjustment to subsequent stressors (Manning & Bouchard, 2020). As society continues to move along the path toward recovering from the COVID-19 pandemic, resource gains in response to place attachment disruption experiences could become sources of strength that enable people to emerge more resilient on the other side of the public health crisis.

References

Blustein, D. L., Duffy, R., Ferreira, J. A., Cohen-Scali, V., Cinamon, R. G., & Allan, B. A. (2020). Unemployment in the time of COVID-19: A research agenda. *Journal of Vocational Behavior, 119*, 103436. https://doi.org/10.1016/j.jvb.2020.103436

Boğaç, C. (2009). Place attachment in a foreign settlement. *Journal of Environmental Psychology, 29*(2), 267–278. https://doi.org/10.1016/j.jenvp.2009.01.001

Brown, B. B., & Perkins, D. D. (1992). Disruptions in place attachment. In I. Altman & S. M. Low (Eds.), *Place attachment* (pp. 279–304). Springer. https://doi.org/10.1007/978-1-4684-8753-4_13

Counted, V. (2018). The Circle of Place Spirituality (CoPS): Towards an attachment and exploration motivational systems approach in the psychology of religion. In A. Village & R. W. Hood (Eds.), *Research in the social scientific study of religion* (Vol. 29, pp. 145–174). Brill. https://doi.org/10.1163/9789004382640_009

Counted, V., Neff, M. A., Captari, L. E., & Cowden, R. G. (2021). Transcending place attachment disruptions during a public health crisis: Spiritual struggles, resilience, and transformation. *Journal of Psychology and Christianity, 39*(4), 276–286.

Counted, V., Pargament, K. I., Bechara, A. O., Joynt, S., & Cowden, R. G. (2020). Hope and well-being in vulnerable contexts during the COVID-19 pandemic: Does religious coping matter? *The Journal of Positive Psychology*. Advance online publication. https://doi.org/10.1080/17439760.2020.1832247

Cowden, R. G., Tucker, L. A., & Govender, K. (2020). Conceptual pathways to HIV risk in Eastern and Southern Africa: An integrative perspective on the development of young people in contexts of social-structural vulnerability. In K. Govender & N. K. Poku (Eds.), *Preventing HIV among young people in Southern and Eastern Africa: Emerging evidence and intervention strategies* (pp. 31–47). Routledge.

Cowden, R. G., Davis, E. B., Counted, V., Chen, Y., Rueger, S. Y., VanderWeele, T. J., Lemke, A. W., Glowiak, K. J., & Worthington, E. L., Jr. (2021). Suffering, mental health, and psychological well-being during the COVID-19 pandemic: A longitudinal study of U.S. adults with chronic health conditions. *Wellbeing, Space and Society, 2*, 100048. https://doi.org/10.1016/j.wss.2021.100048

Cowden, R. G., Rueger, S. Y., Davis, E. B., Counted, V., Kent, B. V., Chen, Y., VanderWeele, T. J., Rim, M., Lemke, A. W., & Worthington, E. L., Jr. (2021). Resource loss, positive religious coping, and suffering during the COVID-19 pandemic: A prospective cohort study of U.S. adults with chronic illness. *Mental Health, Religion & Culture*. Advance online publication. https://doi.org/10.1080/13674676.2021.1948000

Cowden, R. G., Pargament, K. I., Chen, Z. J., Davis, E. B., Lemke, A. W., Glowiak, K. J., Rueger, S. Y., & Worthington, E. L., Jr. (2021). Religious/spiritual struggles and psychological distress: A test of three models in a longitudinal study of adults with chronic health conditions. *Journal of Clinical Psychology*. Advance online publication. https://doi.org/10.1002/jclp.23232

Dein, S., Loewenthal, K., Lewis, C. A., & Pargament, K. I. (2020). COVID-19, mental health and religion: An agenda for future research. *Mental Health, Religion & Culture, 23*(1), 1–9. https://doi.org/10.1080/13674676.2020.1768725

Doane, L. S., Schumm, J. A., & Hobfoll, S. E. (2012). The positive, sustaining, and protective power of resources: Insights from conservation of resources theory. In K. Törnblom & A. Kazemi (Eds.), *Handbook of social resource theory: Theoretical extensions, empirical insights, and social applications* (pp. 301–310). Springer. https://doi.org/10.1007/978-1-4614-4175-5_19

Exline, J. J. (2013). Religious and spiritual struggles. In K. I. Pargament, J. J. Exline, & J. W. Jones (Eds.), *APA handbook of psychology, religion, and spirituality (Vol. 1): Context, theory, and research* (pp. 459–475). American Psychological Association. https://doi.org/10.1037/14045-000

Fredrickson, B. L. (2002). How does religion benefit health and well-being? Are positive emotions active ingredients? *Psychological Inquiry, 13*(3), 209–213.

Govender, K., Cowden, R. G., Nyamaruze, P., Armstrong, R. M., & Hatane, L. (2020). Beyond the disease: Contextualized implications of the COVID-19 pandemic for children and young people living in Eastern and Southern Africa. *Frontiers in Public Health, 8*, 504. https://doi.org/10.3389/fpubh.2020.00504

Halbesleben, J. R. B., Neveu, J.-P., Paustian-Underdahl, S. C., & Westman, M. (2014). Getting to the "COR": Understanding the role of resources in conservation of resources theory. *Journal of Management, 40*(5), 1334–1364. https://doi.org/10.1177/0149206314527130

Hobfoll, S. E. (1989). Conservation of resources: A new attempt at conceptualizing stress. *American Psychologist, 44*(3), 513–524. https://doi.org/10.1037/0003-066X.44.3.513

Hobfoll, S. E. (2001). The influence of culture, community, and the nested-self in the stress process: Advancing Conservation of Resources theory. *Applied Psychology: An International Review, 50*(3), 337–370. https://doi.org/10.1111/1464-0597.00062

Hobfoll, S. E. (2002). Social and psychological resources and adaptation. *Review of General Psychology, 6*(4), 307–324. https://doi.org/10.1037/1089-2680.6.4.307

Hobfoll, S. E., Halbesleben, J., Neveu, J.-P., & Westman, M. (2018). Conservation of resources in the organizational context: The reality of resources and their consequences. *Annual Review of Organizational Psychology and Organizational Behavior, 5*(1), 103–128. https://doi.org/10.1146/annurev-orgpsych-032117-104640

Hobfoll, S. E., & Schumm, J. A. (2009). Conservation of resources theory: Application to public health promotion. In R. J. DiClemente, R. A. Crosby, & M. C. Kegler (Eds.), *Emerging theories in health promotion practice and research* (2nd ed., pp. 131–156). Jossey-Bass.

Hobfoll, S. E., Tirone, V., Holmgreen, L., & Gerhart, J. (2016). Conservation of resources theory applied to major stress. In G. Fink (Ed.), *Stress: Concepts, cognition, emotion, and behavior* (pp. 65–71). Academic. https://doi.org/10.1016/B978-0-12-800951-2.00007-8

Holmgreen, L., Tirone, V., Gerhart, J., & Hobfoll, S. E. (2017). Conservation of resources theory: Resource caravans and passageways in health contexts. In C. L. Cooper & J. C. Quick (Eds.), *The handbook of stress and health: A guide to research and practice* (pp. 443–457). Wiley. https://doi.org/10.1002/9781118993811.ch27

Manning, L. K. (2013). Navigating hardships in old age: Exploring the relationship between spirituality and resilience in later life. *Qualitative Health Research, 23*(4), 568–575. https://doi.org/10.1177/1049732312471730

Manning, L. K., & Bouchard, L. (2020). Encounters with adversity: A framework for understanding resilience in later life. *Aging & Mental Health, 24*(7), 1108–1115. https://doi.org/10.1080/13607863.2019.1594162

O'Connor, R. C., Wetherall, K., Cleare, S., McClelland, H., Melson, A. J., Niedzwiedz, C. L., O'Carroll, R. E., O'Connor, D. B., Platt, S., Scowcroft, E., Watson, B., Zortea, T., Ferguson, E., & Robb, K. A. (2020). Mental health and well-being during the COVID-19 pandemic: Longitudinal analyses of adults in the UK COVID-19 Mental Health & Wellbeing study. *The British Journal of Psychiatry*, 1–8. https://doi.org/10.1192/bjp.2020.212

Pargament, K. I. (1997). *The psychology of religion and coping: Theory, research, practice*. Guilford Press.

Pargament, K. I. (2007). *Spiritually integrated psychotherapy: Understanding and addressing the sacred*. Guilford Press.

Pargament, K. I., & Ano, G. G. (2006). Spiritual resources and struggles in coping with medical illness. *Southern Medical Journal, 99*(10), 1161–1162. https://doi.org/10.1097/01.smj.0000242847.40214.b6

Pargament, K. I., Desai, K. M., & McConnell, K. M. (2006). Spirituality: A pathway to posttraumatic growth or decline? In L. G. Calhoun & R. G. Tedeschi (Eds.), *Handbook of posttraumatic growth: Research & practice* (pp. 121–137). Lawrence Erlbaum Associates.

Pargament, K. I., & Lomax, J. W. (2013). Understanding and addressing religion among people with mental illness. *World Psychiatry, 12*(1), 26–32. https://doi.org/10.1002/wps.20005

Pew Research Center. (2020). *Americans oppose religious exemptions from coronavirus-related restrictions*. Pew Research Center. Retrieved from https://www.pewforum.org/2020/08/07/attending-and-watching-religious-services-in-the-age-of-the-coronavirus/

Ranney, R. M., Bruehlman-Senecal, E., & Ayduk, O. (2017). Comparing the effects of three online cognitive reappraisal trainings on well-being. *Journal of Happiness Studies, 18*(5), 1319–1338. https://doi.org/10.1007/s10902-016-9779-0

Scannell, L., Cox, R. S., Fletcher, S., & Heykoop, C. (2016). "That was the last time I saw my house": The importance of place attachment among children and youth in disaster contexts. *American Journal of Community Psychology, 58*(1–2), 158–173. https://doi.org/10.1002/ajcp.12069

Scannell, L., & Gifford, R. (2017). The experienced psychological benefits of place attachment. *Journal of Environmental Psychology, 51*, 256–269. https://doi.org/10.1016/j.jenvp.2017.04.001

Scannell, L., Williams, E., Gifford, R., & Sarich, C. (2021). Parallels between interpersonal and place attachment: An update. In L. C. Manzo & P. Devine-Wright (Eds.), *Place attachment: Advances in theory, methods, and applications* (2nd ed., pp. 45–60). Routledge.

Shaw, A., Joseph, S., & Linley, P. A. (2005). Religion, spirituality, and posttraumatic growth: A systematic review. *Mental Health, Religion & Culture, 8*(1), 1–11. https://doi.org/10.1080/1367467032000157981

VanderWeele, T. J. (2020). Love of neighbor during a pandemic: Navigating the competing goods of religious gatherings and physical health. *Journal of Religion and Health, 59*(5), 2196–2202. https://doi.org/10.1007/s10943-020-01031-6

Wong, S., Pargament, K. I., & Faigin, C. A. (2018). Sustained by the sacred: Religious and spiritual factors for resilience in adulthood and aging. In B. Resnick, L. P. Gwyther, & K. A. Roberto (Eds.), *Resilience in aging: Concepts, research, and outcomes* (pp. 191–214). Springer. https://doi.org/10.1007/978-3-030-04555-5_10

Xiong, J., Lipsitz, O., Nasri, F., Lui, L. M. W., Gill, H., Phan, L., Chen-Li, D., Iacobucci, M., Ho, R., Majeed, A., & McIntyre, R. S. (2020). Impact of COVID-19 pandemic on mental health in the general population: A systematic review. *Journal of Affective Disorders, 277*, 55–64. https://doi.org/10.1016/j.jad.2020.08.001

Zhang, S. X., Wang, Y., Rauch, A., & Wei, F. (2020). Unprecedented disruption of lives and work: Health, distress and life satisfaction of working adults in China one month into the COVID-19 outbreak. *Psychiatry Research, 288*, 112958. https://doi.org/10.1016/j.psychres.2020.112958

Chapter 7
Transcending Place Attachment Disruption: Strengthening Character During a Pandemic

Richard G. Cowden, Victor Counted, and Haywantee Ramkissoon

Contents

Virtues and Character Strengths..	82
Pathways to Transcending Place Attachment Disruption: Gratitude, Hope, and Spirituality....	83
Gratitude..	84
Hope..	85
Spirituality...	87
Conclusion...	88
References..	88

In Chapters 3 and 6, we discussed the principle that people are naturally driven to invest resources in order to regain, restore, or rebound from resource loss (Hobfoll, 2012). Attempts at offsetting resource loss can take different forms, most of which are functionally adaptive in that they are employed as means of dealing with the challenges a person encounters (Holmgreen et al., 2017). However, the consequences of how a person responds to loss can vary on a spectrum ranging from adaptive to maladaptive. A functionally adaptive approach to recovering from a loss might be useful in the short-term, but it could have unfavorable long-term implications for health and well-being (Wadsworth, 2015). Resource investment responses that balance both short- and long-term ideals may be particularly useful for dealing with resource loss in a way that promotes a more enduring level of positive adjustment.

This chapter provides an overview of how resource loss that accompanies place attachment disruption during the COVID-19 pandemic might be transformed into a character-building process that supports short-term adaptation and long-term well-being. Using the virtue of *transcendence* as a framework (Peterson & Seligman, 2004), it considers three interconnected character strengths—gratitude, hope, and spirituality—that can support exploration and integration of past, present, and future experiences connected to a place of attachment that has been disrupted by the public health crisis. It also outlines some targeted activities that engage each of these transcendent character strengths, the benefits of which could facilitate sustainable adjustment to pandemic-related place attachment disruption experiences and enable people to recover more quickly in the aftermath of the COVID-19 pandemic.

Virtues and Character Strengths

Around the time that positive psychology emerged as a mainstream subfield of psychology, Dahlsgaard et al. (2005) conducted a landmark study to identify a universal set of valued human strengths. Their review of foundational texts from major philosophical (e.g., Athenian philosophy) and religious traditions (e.g., Buddhism) around the world revealed six superordinate constituents of *good character* that are common across cultures, belief systems, and history: courage, humanity, justice, temperance, transcendence, and wisdom. They referred to these abstract principles of socially desirable functioning as core virtues (McGrath et al., 2018). As general dimensions of positive social functioning, the virtues are thought to be appreciable to the extent that a person displays an underlying collection of character strengths. The six virtues have been used as higher-order categories in a hierarchical model that includes 24 lower-order character strengths, each of which corresponds to one of the six virtues (Peterson & Seligman, 2004). Each character strength is understood as a relatively stable personality characteristic (Niemiec, 2013), but the enduring quality of character strengths does not imply that they are fixed and cannot be developed or improved (Park & Peterson, 2008). A growing body of empirical literature indicates that character strengths can be cultivated through interventions that encourage people to apply character strengths in their daily lives (Ruch et al., 2020).

Character strengths have several features that make them attractive as resources for people who have experienced place attachment disruption during the COVID-19 pandemic. First, character strengths serve self-regulatory functions that enable people to cope effectively with adversity (Martínez-Martí & Ruch, 2017; Peterson et al., 2008). Resource loss that underlies place attachment disruption during the COVID-19 pandemic will vary, but character strengths could equip people with a repertoire of capacities that empower them to respond adaptively to a range of losses. For example, many intangible losses associated with place attachment disruption experiences (e.g., sense of peace) could be addressed by accessing the self-regulatory mechanisms (e.g., meaning-making) of particular character strengths. Numerous studies have reported on the effectiveness of character strength interventions in reducing psychological distress and improving subjective well-being (for reviews, see Quinlan et al., 2012; Yan et al., 2020; for a meta-analysis, see Schutte & Malouff, 2019). Although the self-regulatory functions of character strengths may be oriented principally toward bringing about benefits in the short-term, character strength development in response to pandemic-related place attachment disruption could also support positive adjustment in the longer-term as people are confronted with other forms of resource loss over time.

Second, a fundamental criterion of character strengths is that they contribute to fulfilling constituents that make up "the good life" (Peterson & Seligman, 2004). In times of crisis, character strengths can direct a person's attention toward evaluating the quality of their life pursuits. The discomfort of being separated from a place of attachment could represent an opportune time for re-evaluating activities, goals, and priorities because the place of attachment and its accompanying benefits are no longer able to fulfill the needs they formerly did (Counted et al., 2021). Through character strengths, renewed energies might be dedicated to finding alternative avenues to fulfill meaningful life pursuits that were prioritized before pandemic-related place attachment disruption transpired (e.g., relationship with the sacred). On the other hand, character strengths might lead to a person who has been separated from a place of attachment to prioritize meaningful life pursuits that were previously underemphasized, neglected, or overlooked entirely.

Pathways to Transcending Place Attachment Disruption: Gratitude, Hope, and Spirituality

Character strengths are viewed as a set of psychological ingredients that collectively contribute to living a fulfilled life. However, situational demands may require that some character strengths be emphasized over others (Biswas-Diener et al., 2011; Niemiec, 2013). One subset of character strengths that may be particularly useful to people who are dealing with pandemic-related place attachment disruption includes gratitude, hope, and spirituality, which are classified under the virtue of transcendence (Van Cappellen & Rimé, 2014). This trio of character strengths supports adaptive cognitive-emotional processing of subjective experiences by connecting people with memories from the past, present experiences, and future potentialities. Together, gratitude, hope, and spirituality provide people with opportunities to look beyond the demands of their current circumstances, facilitate meaning-making, and cultivate a sense of connection to the larger universe (Peterson & Seligman, 2004). Those generative experiences could transform the challenges of pandemic-related place attachment disruption into pathways that lead to psychospiritual resilience and character development.

Although the following sections describe the potential value of gratitude, hope, and spirituality in supporting people who have experienced pandemic-related place attachment disruption, it is important to mention that the significance of these character strengths comes from their interrelatedness. Some research indicates that gratitude, hope, and spirituality tend to develop alongside one another (Peterson & Seligman, 2003). A number of studies have found that gratitude, hope, and spirituality are at least moderately associated with each other (e.g., Marques et al., 2013; McCullough et al., 2004; Witvliet et al., 2019, Study 1). Other evidence suggests that gains in these strengths can contribute to improvements in one another. For example, spirituality has been shown to predict positive changes in gratitude (Olson et al., 2019), and practicing gratitude can promote hope (Witvliet et al., 2019, Study 2). Hence, gratitude, hope, and spirituality could have the most powerful implications for those who have been separated from a place of attachment during the COVID-19 pandemic when they are understood and applied as a network of transcendent character strengths.

Gratitude

Gratitude broadly involves recognizing and appreciating the positive in life (Wood et al., 2010). Like other affective phenomena, the psychological constituents of gratitude intersect trait, mood, and emotion levels of affective experience (McCullough et al., 2004). As a trait, gratitude can be understood as a disposition toward experiencing grateful emotions in response to personally beneficial life experiences and outcomes (Portocarrero et al., 2020). A grateful disposition lowers a person's threshold for experiencing grateful emotions (McCullough et al., 2002). In an intermediate territory wedged between the trait and emotion levels of affective experience, gratitude has also been identified as a stable positive mood that can have subtle but pervasive effects on consciousness for relatively long periods of time (McCullough et al., 2004). At the emotional level, gratitude refers to an acute, intense, and momentary psychophysiological response that arises when a person notices and appreciates the positive in a particular aspect of their lived experience (Emmons et al., 2019). Although the trait, mood, and emotion levels of gratitude have distinct properties, they are interrelated. For example, research has found that grateful moods manifest through additive and interactive top-down (i.e., trait) and bottom-up (i.e., emotion) effects (McCullough et al., 2004).

Numerous observational and experimental studies have found that gratitude is associated with many indices of well-being, promotes positive psychosocial functioning, and protects against the negative effects of adverse circumstances (for a review, see Wood et al., 2010; for meta-analysis, see Dickens, 2017). The benefits of gratitude can be traced to self-regulatory cognitive processes (e.g., contrasting, positive reframing, savoring) that direct a person's attention toward "the good" (Alkozei et al., 2018; Lambert, Graham, et al., 2009; Wood et al., 2008). By harnessing the cognitive processes that underpin gratitude, people who are grappling with the effects of pandemic-related place attachment disruption might find respite through the pleasant experience of gratitude. To illustrate, a person could approach their experience of place attachment disruption by identifying the ways in which their situation compares more favorably to the extent of loss that they have experienced in the past (i.e., contrasting). Alternatively, a person might focus on identifying the positive features of their challenging circumstances (i.e., positive reframing). A person could also reflect upon positive past experiences that are connected to the place of attachment they have been separated from (i.e., savoring). These kinds of cognitive processes represent some of the pathways to experiencing gratitude (Emmons & Mishra, 2011), many of which form part of interventions that have been developed to promote gratitude.

The most widely used approaches to increase gratitude include written exercises (e.g., gratitude journaling), behavioral expressions of gratitude (e.g., sending letters of gratitude to others), and grateful contemplation (e.g., guided gratitude meditation). Research suggests that gratitude interventions are effective at reducing psychological distress and improving subjective well-being in a wide range of populations (Emmons & Stern, 2013; Lomas et al., 2014). Beyond the psychological benefits that accompany gratitude interventions, several studies have found that gratitude activities also produce positive changes at both mood and disposition levels of gratitude (Dickens, 2017). Those findings are noteworthy because they suggest that there is potential to increase the pervasiveness of gratitude in a person's day-to-day life. If people who have encountered pandemic-related place attachment disruption are able to consistently increase their experience of grateful emotions over the short-term, gratitude could develop into an enduring psychological resource that becomes useful when future resource loss occurs. More generally, broaden-and-build theory suggests that increasing grateful emotions through targeted activities might contribute to building other resources (e.g., social bonds, spirituality) that a person can draw on to successfully deal with subsequent adversity (Fredrickson, 2004).

Hope

Hope can be defined as an orientation toward the possibility of a future good outcome with a desire that has the strength to overcome challenges (Sain, 2020). Similar to historical conceptions of hope, empirical research suggests that the salient principles of hope are that the object of hope is morally acceptable and perceived as important, the outcome is realistic but difficult to attain, and the person is willing to take appropriate steps to achieve the desired outcome (Averill et al., 1990). Research within positive psychology has been dominated by cognitive-motivational perspectives in which hope is described as a motivational force that is anchored in goals or the pursuit of positive outcomes (Scioli, 2020).

One of the most popular models of hope is Snyder's (2000, 2002) goal-focused theory, which asserts that hope centers on a person's motivation to pursue goal-directed behavior (i.e., willpower) and their capacity to identify pathways to achieving those goals (i.e., waypower). However, evidence suggests that goal attainment may only be a minor component of hope in some settings (Larsen & Stege, 2012). For example, research has found that hope can be experienced as an emotion that arises when a person is focused on a positive outcome (Bruininks & Malle, 2005). Yet the emotional component of hope tends to be underemphasized in popular cognitive-motivational theories of the concept. In fact, the emotional qualities of hope may play a key role in initiating (Lazarus, 1999) and sustaining (Averill et al., 1990) a person's pursuit of a future outcome. These complexities have led to the development of integrative theoretical frameworks that attempt to capture hope more comprehensively. For example, Scioli et al. (2011) conceptualized hope as a self-regulatory network comprising four interrelated biopsychospiritual constituents—mastery, attachment, survival, and spirituality—rooted in a five-level developmental structure. An important feature of this and other integrative frameworks (e.g., Ward & Wampler, 2010) is that they accommodate a wide range of potential objects of hope and a variety of sources that could facilitate the development and maintenance of hope.

An abundance of research indicates that hope is positively associated with improved mental health, physical health, and positive psychosocial functioning (for reviews, see Gallagher & Lopez, 2018). Consistent with theoretical accounts that highlight the centrality of hope in the coping process (e.g., Folkman, 2013), studies have found that hope may protect against the negative effects of adversity on psychological well-being (see Gallagher et al., 2020). Similar findings have emerged in research on the COVID-19 pandemic (Counted et al., 2020; Gallagher et al., 2021), suggesting that hope could be a useful psychological resource for people who are navigating the difficulties associated with pandemic-related place attachment disruption.

The most common approaches to building hope are grounded in Snyder's hope theory (see Gallagher & Lopez, 2018). The basic components of interventions that apply this goal-focused theory include identifying a meaningful goal, fostering positive thoughts about personal agency, and generating multiple pathways that could be pursued to achieve the desired goal. This framework could prove useful for many people in pursuit of a goal that is tethered to a place of attachment that they have been separated from during the COVID-19 pandemic. For example, a person may rediscover the value of maintaining hopeful thoughts and find renewed goal-oriented motivation by reflecting on events in the past where obstacles and setbacks were overcome on the way to achieving a particular goal.

Psychological intervention research indicates that goal-oriented hope enhancement strategies have the potential to increase hope and subjective well-being (for a meta-analysis, see Weis & Speridakos, 2011). However, approaches that focus on goals alone may have limited effectiveness in supporting people who are experiencing psychological distress in response to pandemic-related place attachment disruption, in part because opportunities to pursue certain goals have been thwarted by many factors that were outside of one's personal control (e.g., stay-at-home orders). Depending on the object of a person's hope, alternative resource investment strategies might be better suited to fostering hope among those who have been separated from a place of attachment during the COVID-19 pandemic. For example, research has found that hope can be promoted by social support (Xiang et al., 2020), including support derived from groups or communities composed of people who share similar life experiences (Schrank et al., 2008).

Within the context of the COVID-19 pandemic, online communities that bring together those struggling with place attachment disruption could facilitate transformational experiences (e.g., a shared sense of meaning) that contribute to restoring or sustaining hope. For some people, pandemic-related place attachment disruption might be an opportunity to shift their hope toward an object that supports the development of a persistent and resolute hope. Compared to an object of hope that is organized around achieving a specific outcome, those who invest in hope that is oriented toward mastery (e.g., seeking new experiences, having a sense of purpose in life) may develop a hope that is liberating, empowering, and can transcend worldly challenges that often bring about feelings of hopelessness.

Spirituality

Spirituality is a complex, multidimensional concept (Schlehofer et al., 2008). At its core, spirituality has been described as a dynamic process that involves searching for and connecting with God, the divine, or a transcendent reality (Pargament, 1999). It is considered an irreducible motivational force that shapes, guides, and maintains growth-oriented pursuits that center on engaging with and becoming closer to the sacred (Lomas, 2019; Pargament, 2013). Spirituality has the potential to permeate across life domains (Hill et al., 2000) and to integrate all dimensions of the human experience to promote optimal well-being (Chandler et al., 1992).

Various dimensions of spirituality (e.g., beliefs, faith, activities) are associated with improved mental health and subjective well-being (for reviews, see Braam & Koenig, 2019; Hardy et al., 2019; for a meta-analysis, see Garssen et al., 2021). When people experience crises, spirituality often becomes part of the resources they draw on to cope (Harper & Pargament, 2015). Although spirituality may not offer solutions to all forms of resource loss, research has found that spirituality functions as a source of resilience and buffers the impact of stressors on well-being (Gall & Guirguis-Younger, 2013). For those grappling with resource loss that underlies place attachment disruption during the COVID-19 pandemic, spirituality could be an invaluable resource that facilitates immediate and long-term positive adjustment. For example, spirituality can provide people who have experienced place attachment disruption with a framework for finding meaning in their situation and maintaining a sense of purpose amid hardship (Counted et al., 2021). Spirituality might also become an essential part of how people transform their experience of place attachment disruption into an adaptive process that culminates in the formation of new attachment bonds (i.e., detachment).

Pandemic-related place attachment disruption presents an opportunity for people to develop a richer understanding of the sacred, a deeper level of intimacy with the divine, and move closer toward self-transcendence. Progress toward those ends can be achieved through spiritual disciplines (e.g., prayer, reading scripture, meditation), which are undertaken to generate spiritual experiences (e.g., felt presence of the sacred). Some evidence indicates that engaging in spiritual disciplines can reduce psychological distress. For example, many studies have reported evidence supporting the effectiveness of mindfulness meditation in improving anxiety and depression (for a meta-analysis, see Goyal et al., 2014). However, the implications of investing in spiritual disciplines may be far more extensive for people who have been confronted with place attachment disruption during the COVID-19 pandemic. Specifically, spiritual disciplines promote spiritual development and often become an important part of a person's journey toward spiritual maturity (Gallagher & Newton, 2009). They also cultivate other character strengths (including gratitude and hope) that contribute to personal growth (Lambert, Fincham, et al., 2009; Munoz et al., 2016). Over time, spiritual disciplines could lead to a reservoir of psychospiritual resources that support long-term resilience and well-being in the face of future resource loss (Agarwal et al., 2020).

Conclusion

Successful adaptation to resource loss that accompanies place attachment disruption during the COVID-19 pandemic requires a resource investment response that balances short-term recovery and long-term well-being. This chapter provided an overview of gratitude, hope, and spirituality as three transcendent character strengths that people who have been separated from a place of attachment could mobilize to build the kind of psychospiritual resources that enable them to deal with current and future resource loss. Although there will always be resource loss that cannot be completely offset by character strengths alone, people who are able to harness and pursue gratitude, hope, and spirituality may develop a set of psychospiritual resources that facilitate positive adjustment and contribute more broadly to self-actualization.

References

Agarwal, K., Fortune, L., Heintzman, J. C., & Kelly, L. L. (2020). Spiritual experiences of long-term meditation practitioners diagnosed with breast cancer: An interpretative phenomenological analysis pilot study. *Journal of Religion and Health, 59*(5), 2364–2380. https://doi.org/10.1007/s10943-020-00995-9

Alkozei, A., Smith, R., & Killgore, W. D. S. (2018). Gratitude and subjective wellbeing: A proposal of two causal frameworks. *Journal of Happiness Studies, 19*(5), 1519–1542. https://doi.org/10.1007/s10902-017-9870-1

Averill, J. R., Catlin, G., & Chon, K. K. (1990). Study 1: The anatomy of hope. In J. R. Averill, G. Catlin, & K. K. Chon (Eds.), *Rules of hope* (pp. 9–35). Springer. https://doi.org/10.1007/978-1-4613-9674-1_2

Biswas-Diener, R., Kashdan, T. B., & Minhas, G. (2011). A dynamic approach to psychological strength development and intervention. *The Journal of Positive Psychology, 6*(2), 106–118. https://doi.org/10.1080/17439760.2010.545429

Braam, A. W., & Koenig, H. G. (2019). Religion, spirituality and depression in prospective studies: A systematic review. *Journal of Affective Disorders, 257*, 428–438. https://doi.org/10.1016/j.jad.2019.06.063

Bruininks, P., & Malle, B. F. (2005). Distinguishing hope from optimism and related affective states. *Motivation and Emotion, 29*(4), 324–352. https://doi.org/10.1007/s11031-006-9010-4

Chandler, C. K., Holden, J. M., & Kolander, C. A. (1992). Counseling for spiritual wellness: Theory and practice. *Journal of Counseling & Development, 71*(2), 168–175. https://doi.org/10.1002/j.1556-6676.1992.tb02193.x

Counted, V., Neff, M. A., Captari, L. E., & Cowden, R. G. (2021). Transcending place attachment disruptions during a public health crisis: Spiritual struggles, resilience, and transformation. *Journal of Psychology and Christianity, 39*(4), 276–286.

Counted, V., Pargament, K. I., Bechara, A. O., Joynt, S., & Cowden, R. G. (2020). Hope and well-being in vulnerable contexts during the COVID-19 pandemic: Does religious coping matter? *The Journal of Positive Psychology.* Advance online publication. https://doi.org/10.1080/17439760.2020.1832247

Dahlsgaard, K., Peterson, C., & Seligman, M. E. P. (2005). Shared virtue: The convergence of valued human strengths across culture and history. *Review of General Psychology, 9*(3), 203–213. https://doi.org/10.1037/1089-2680.9.3.203

Dickens, L. R. (2017). Using gratitude to promote positive change: A series of meta-analyses investigating the effectiveness of gratitude interventions. *Basic and Applied Social Psychology, 39*(4), 193–208. https://doi.org/10.1080/01973533.2017.1323638

Emmons, R. A., Froh, J., & Rose, R. (2019). Gratitude. In M. W. Gallagher & S. J. Lopez (Eds.), *Positive psychological assessment: A handbook of models and measures* (2nd ed., pp. 317–332). American Psychological Association. https://doi.org/10.1037/0000138-020

Emmons, R. A., & Mishra, A. (2011). Why gratitude enhances well-being: What we know, what we need to know. In K. M. Sheldon, T. B. Kashdan, & M. F. Steger (Eds.), *Designing positive psychology: Taking stock and moving forward* (pp. 248–262). Oxford University Press. https://doi.org/10.1093/acprof:oso/9780195373585.003.0016

Emmons, R. A., & Stern, R. (2013). Gratitude as a psychotherapeutic intervention. *Journal of Clinical Psychology, 69*(8), 846–855. https://doi.org/10.1002/jclp.22020

Folkman, S. (2013). Stress, coping, and hope. In B. I. Carr & J. Steel (Eds.), *Psychological aspects of cancer* (pp. 119–127). Springer. https://doi.org/10.1007/978-1-4614-4866-2_8

Fredrickson, B. L. (2004). Gratitude, like other positive emotions, broadens and builds. In R. A. Emmons & M. E. McCullough (Eds.), *The psychology of gratitude* (pp. 145–166). Oxford University Press. https://doi.org/10.1093/acprof:oso/9780195150100.003.0008

Gall, T. L., & Guirguis-Younger, M. (2013). Religious and spiritual coping: Current theory and research. In K. I. Pargament, J. J. Exline, & J. W. Jones (Eds.), *APA handbook of psychology, religion, and spirituality (Vol. 1): Context, theory, and research* (pp. 349–364). American Psychological Association. https://doi.org/10.1037/14045-019

Gallagher, M. W., Long, L. J., & Phillips, C. A. (2020). Hope, optimism, self-efficacy, and post-traumatic stress disorder: A meta-analytic review of the protective effects of positive expectancies. *Journal of Clinical Psychology, 76*(3), 329–355. https://doi.org/10.1002/jclp.22882

Gallagher, M. W., & Lopez, S. J. (2018). *The Oxford handbook of hope.* Oxford University Press.

Gallagher, M. W., Smith, L. J., Richardson, A. L., D'Souza, J. M., & Long, L. J. (2021). Examining the longitudinal effects and potential mechanisms of hope on COVID-19 stress, anxiety, and well-being. *Cognitive Behaviour Therapy.* Advance online publication. https://doi.org/10.1080/16506073.2021.1877341

Gallagher, S. K., & Newton, C. (2009). Defining spiritual growth: Congregations, community, and connectedness. *Sociology of Religion, 70*(3), 232–261. https://doi.org/10.1093/socrel/srp039

Garssen, B., Visser, A., & Pool, G. (2021). Does spirituality or religion positively affect mental health? Meta-analysis of longitudinal studies. *The International Journal for the Psychology of Religion, 31*(1), 4–20. https://doi.org/10.1080/10508619.2020.1729570

Goyal, M., Singh, S., Sibinga, E. M. S., Gould, N. F., Rowland-Seymour, A., Sharma, R., Berger, Z., Sleicher, D., Maron, D. D., Shihab, H. M., Ranasinghe, P. D., Linn, S., Saha, S., Bass, E. B., & Haythornthwaite, J. A. (2014). Meditation programs for psychological stress and well-being: A systematic review and meta-analysis. *JAMA Internal Medicine, 174*(3), 357–368. https://doi.org/10.1001/jamainternmed.2013.13018

Hardy, S. A., Nelson, J. M., Moore, J. P., & King, P. E. (2019). Processes of religious and spiritual influence in adolescence: A systematic review of 30 years of research. *Journal of Research on Adolescence, 29*(2), 254–275. https://doi.org/10.1111/jora.12486

Harper, A. R., & Pargament, K. I. (2015). Trauma, religion, and spirituality: Pathways to healing. In K. E. Cherry (Ed.), *Traumatic stress and long-term recovery: Coping with disasters and other negative life events* (pp. 349–367). Springer. https://doi.org/10.1007/978-3-319-18866-9_19

Hill, P. C., Pargament, K. I., Hood, R. W., McCullough, M. E., Jr., Swyers, J. P., Larson, D. B., & Zinnbauer, B. J. (2000). Conceptualizing religion and spirituality: Points of commonality, points of departure. *Journal for the Theory of Social Behaviour, 30*(1), 51–77. https://doi.org/10.1111/1468-5914.00119

Hobfoll, S. E. (2012). Conservation of resources and disaster in cultural context: The caravans and passageways for resources. *Psychiatry: Interpersonal and Biological Processes, 75*(3), 227–232. https://doi.org/10.1521/psyc.2012.75.3.227

Holmgreen, L., Tirone, V., Gerhart, J., & Hobfoll, S. E. (2017). Conservation of resources theory: Resource caravans and passageways in health contexts. In C. L. Cooper & J. C. Quick (Eds.), *The handbook of stress and health: A guide to research and practice* (pp. 443–457). Wiley. https://doi.org/10.1002/9781118993811.ch27

Lambert, N. M., Fincham, F. D., Braithwaite, S. R., Graham, S. M., & Beach, S. R. H. (2009). Can prayer increase gratitude? *Psychology of Religion and Spirituality, 1*(3), 139–149. https://doi.org/10.1037/a0016731

Lambert, N. M., Graham, S. M., Fincham, F. D., & Stillman, T. F. (2009). A changed perspective: How gratitude can affect sense of coherence through positive reframing. *The Journal of Positive Psychology, 4*(6), 461–470. https://doi.org/10.1080/17439760903157182

Larsen, D. J., & Stege, R. (2012). Client accounts of hope in early counseling sessions: A qualitative study. *Journal of Counseling & Development, 90*(1), 45–54. https://doi.org/10.1111/j.1556-6676.2012.00007.x

Lazarus, R. S. (1999). Hope: An emotion and a vital coping resource against despair. *Social Research, 66*(2), 653–678.

Lomas, T. (2019). The dynamics of spirituality: A cross-cultural lexical analysis. *Psychology of Religion and Spirituality, 11*(2), 131–140. https://doi.org/10.1037/rel0000163

Lomas, T., Froh, J. J., Emmons, R. A., Mishra, A., & Bono, G. (2014). Gratitude interventions: A review and future agenda. In A. C. Parks & S. M. Schueller (Eds.), *The Wiley Blackwell handbook of positive psychological interventions* (pp. 1–19). Wiley. https://doi.org/10.1002/9781118315927.ch1

Marques, S. C., Lopez, S. J., & Mitchell, J. (2013). The role of hope, spirituality and religious practice in adolescents' life satisfaction: Longitudinal findings. *Journal of Happiness Studies, 14*(1), 251–261. https://doi.org/10.1007/s10902-012-9329-3

Martínez-Martí, M. L., & Ruch, W. (2017). Character strengths predict resilience over and above positive affect, self-efficacy, optimism, social support, self-esteem, and life satisfaction. *The Journal of Positive Psychology, 12*(2), 110–119. https://doi.org/10.1080/17439760.2016.1163403

McGrath, R. E., Greenberg, M. J., & Hall-Simmonds, A. (2018). Scarecrow, Tin Woodsman, and Cowardly Lion: The three-factor model of virtue. *The Journal of Positive Psychology, 13*(4), 373–392. https://doi.org/10.1080/17439760.2017.1326518

McCullough, M. E., Emmons, R. A., & Tsang, J.-A. (2002). The grateful disposition: A conceptual and empirical topography. *Journal of Personality and Social Psychology, 82*(1), 112–127. https://doi.org/10.1037/0022-3514.82.1.112

McCullough, M. E., Tsang, J.-A., & Emmons, R. A. (2004). Gratitude in intermediate affective terrain: Links of grateful moods to individual differences and daily emotional experience. *Journal of Personality and Social Psychology, 86*(2), 295–309. https://doi.org/10.1037/0022-3514.86.2.295

Munoz, R. T., Hoppes, S., Hellman, C. M., Brunk, K. L., Bragg, J. E., & Cummins, C. (2016). The effects of mindfulness meditation on hope and stress. *Research on Social Work Practice, 28*(6), 696–707. https://doi.org/10.1177/1049731516674319

Niemiec, R. M. (2013). VIA character strengths: Research and practice (the first 10 years). In H. H. Knoop & A. Delle Fave (Eds.), *Well-being and cultures: Perspectives from positive psychology* (pp. 11–29). Springer. https://doi.org/10.1007/978-94-007-4611-4_2

Olson, R., Knepple Carney, A., & Hicks Patrick, J. (2019). Associations between gratitude and spirituality: An experience sampling approach. *Psychology of Religion and Spirituality, 11*(4), 449–452. https://doi.org/10.1037/rel0000164

Pargament, K. I. (1999). The psychology of religion and spirituality? Yes and no. *International Journal for the Psychology of Religion, 9*(1), 3–16. https://doi.org/10.1207/s15327582ijpr0901_2

Pargament, K. I. (2013). Searching for the sacred: Toward a non-reductionistic theory of spirituality. In K. I. Pargament, J. J. Exline, & J. W. Jones (Eds.), *APA handbook of psychology, religion, and spirituality (Vol. 1): Context, theory, and research* (pp. 257–273). American Psychological Association. https://doi.org/10.1037/14045-014

Park, N., & Peterson, C. (2008). The cultivation of character strengths. In M. Ferrari & G. Potworowski (Eds.), *Teaching for wisdom: Cross-cultural perspectives on fostering wisdom* (pp. 59–77). Springer. https://doi.org/10.1007/978-1-4020-6532-3_4

Peterson, C., Park, N., Pole, N., D'Andrea, W., & Seligman, M. E. P. (2008). Strengths of character and posttraumatic growth. *Journal of Traumatic Stress, 21*(2), 214–217. https://doi.org/10.1002/jts.20332

Peterson, C., & Seligman, M. E. P. (2003). Character strengths before and after September 11. *Psychological Science, 14*(4), 381–384. https://doi.org/10.1111/1467-9280.24482

Peterson, C., & Seligman, M. E. P. (2004). *Character strengths and virtues: A handbook and classification*. American Psychological Association.

Portocarrero, F. F., Gonzalez, K., & Ekema-Agbaw, M. (2020). A meta-analytic review of the relationship between dispositional gratitude and well-being. *Personality and Individual Differences, 164*, 110101. https://doi.org/10.1016/j.paid.2020.110101

Quinlan, D., Swain, N., & Vella-Brodrick, D. A. (2012). Character strengths interventions: Building on what we know for improved outcomes. *Journal of Happiness Studies, 13*(6), 1145–1163. https://doi.org/10.1007/s10902-011-9311-5

Ruch, W., Niemiec, R. M., McGrath, R. E., Gander, F., & Proyer, R. T. (2020). Character strengths-based interventions: Open questions and ideas for future research. *The Journal of Positive Psychology, 15*(5), 680–684. https://doi.org/10.1080/17439760.2020.1789700

Sain, B. (2020). What is this hope?: Insights from Christian theology and positive psychology. *Journal of Moral Theology, 9*(1), 98–119.

Schlehofer, M. M., Omoto, A. M., & Adelman, J. R. (2008). How do "religion" and "spirituality" differ? Lay definitions among older adults. *Journal for the Scientific Study of Religion, 47*(3), 411–425. https://doi.org/10.1111/j.1468-5906.2008.00418.x

Schrank, B., Stanghellini, G., & Slade, M. (2008). Hope in psychiatry: A review of the literature. *Acta Psychiatrica Scandinavica, 118*(6), 421–433. https://doi.org/10.1111/j.1600-0447.2008.01271.x

Schutte, N. S., & Malouff, J. M. (2019). The impact of signature character strengths interventions: A meta-analysis. *Journal of Happiness Studies, 20*(4), 1179–1196. https://doi.org/10.1007/s10902-018-9990-2

Scioli, A. (2020). The psychology of hope: A diagnostic and prescriptive account. In S. C. van den Heuvel (Ed.), *Historical and multidisciplinary perspectives on hope* (pp. 137–163). Springer. https://doi.org/10.1007/978-3-030-46489-9_8

Scioli, A., Ricci, M., Nyugen, T., & Scioli, E. R. (2011). Hope: Its nature and measurement. *Psychology of Religion and Spirituality, 3*(2), 78–97. https://doi.org/10.1037/a0020903

Snyder, C. R. (2000). The past and possible futures of hope. *Journal of Social and Clinical Psychology, 19*(1), 11–28. https://doi.org/10.1521/jscp.2000.19.1.11

Snyder, C. R. (2002). Hope theory: Rainbows in the mind. *Psychological Inquiry, 13*(4), 249–275. https://doi.org/10.1207/S15327965PLI1304_01

Van Cappellen, P., & Rimé, B. (2014). Positive emotions and self-transcendence. In V. Saroglou (Ed.), *Religion, personality, and social behavior* (pp. 123–145). Psychology Press.

Wadsworth, M. E. (2015). Development of maladaptive coping: A functional adaptation to chronic, uncontrollable stress. *Child Development Perspectives, 9*(2), 96–100. https://doi.org/10.1111/cdep.12112

Ward, D. B., & Wampler, K. S. (2010). Moving up the continuum of hope: Developing a theory of hope and understanding its influence in couples therapy. *Journal of Marital and Family Therapy, 36*(2), 212–228. https://doi.org/10.1111/j.1752-0606.2009.00173.x

Weis, R., & Speridakos, E. C. (2011). A meta-analysis of hope enhancement strategies in clinical and community settings. *Psychology of Well-Being: Theory, Research and Practice, 1*, 5. https://doi.org/10.1186/2211-1522-1-5

Witvliet, C. V. O., Richie, F. J., Root Luna, L. M., & Van Tongeren, D. R. (2019). Gratitude predicts hope and happiness: A two-study assessment of traits and states. *The Journal of Positive Psychology, 14*(3), 271–282. https://doi.org/10.1080/17439760.2018.1424924

Wood, A. M., Froh, J. J., & Geraghty, A. W. A. (2010). Gratitude and well-being: A review and theoretical integration. *Positive Clinical Psychology, 30*(7), 890–905. https://doi.org/10.1016/j.cpr.2010.03.005

Wood, A. M., Maltby, J., Stewart, N., Linley, P. A., & Joseph, S. (2008). A social-cognitive model of trait and state levels of gratitude. *Emotion, 8*(2), 281–290. https://doi.org/10.1037/1528-3542.8.2.281

Xiang, G., Teng, Z., Li, Q., Chen, H., & Guo, C. (2020). The influence of perceived social support on hope: A longitudinal study of older-aged adolescents in China. *Children and Youth Services Review, 119*, 105616. https://doi.org/10.1016/j.childyouth.2020.105616

Yan, T., Chan, C. W. H., Chow, K. M., Zheng, W., & Sun, M. (2020). A systematic review of the effects of character strengths-based intervention on the psychological well-being of patients suffering from chronic illnesses. *Journal of Advanced Nursing, 76*(7), 1567–1580. https://doi.org/10.1111/jan.14356

Chapter 8
Pro-environmental Behavior, Place Attachment, and Human Flourishing: Implications for Post-pandemic Research, Theory, Practice, and Policy

Victor Counted, Richard G. Cowden, and Haywantee Ramkissoon

Contents

Pro-environmental Behavior as Planned Behavior.	94
From Pro-environmental Behavior to Place Attachment.	95
Place Attachment and Flourishing.	97
Fostering Place Flourishing After a Pandemic.	99
Identification.	99
Examination.	100
Design.	100
Evaluation.	101
Implications for Theory, Research, Policy, and Practice.	102
Theory.	102
Research.	103
Policy.	104
Practice.	104
Conclusion.	105
References.	105

In earlier chapters, we addressed the impact that the COVID-19 pandemic has had on people-place relationships and some of the avenues that people could pursue to effectively cope with and transcend place attachment disruption experiences. In this chapter, we focus on the potential for place-based experiences to provide people with opportunities to rebuild or develop new attachment relationships with places after the COVID-19 pandemic. Specifically, we explore pro-environmental behavior as a place-based experience that (1) offers people a safe and environmentally friendly opportunity to positively interact with the environment, (2) can foster healthy connections with places and people within places, and (3) contributes more broadly to societal flourishing. Given the extent of displacement and emplacement that has taken place during the COVID-19 pandemic, we suggest that pro-environmental behavior should be emphasized by researchers, healthcare practitioners, and policy makers during the post-pandemic recovery process because it has promising

© The Author(s), under exclusive license to Springer Nature Switzerland AG 2021
V. Counted et al., *Place and Post-Pandemic Flourishing*, SpringerBriefs in Psychology, https://doi.org/10.1007/978-3-030-82580-5_8

potential to promote human flourishing by enhancing place attachment. An equally appealing benefit of pro-environmental behavior is that it can be harnessed to address urgent environmental issues facing society, including climate change, environmental deterioration, and pollution (Di Marco et al., 2020; Reese et al., 2020). In the sections that follow, we expand on these ideas by bringing together principles of planned behavior and place attachment to explore how the Identification, Examination, Design, and Evaluation (IEDE) framework (Steg & Vlek, 2009) could be integrated into research and practice to cultivate pro-environmental behaviors that stimulate the kinds of relationships with place that would enable sustainable human and planetary flourishing after the COVID-19 pandemic.

Pro-environmental Behavior as Planned Behavior

Over the years, several theoretical models have been proposed to capture the antecedents of pro-environmental behavior under a unifying framework. There is some variation in the complexity and components that comprise each of the models that currently exist (for reviews, see Bamberg & Möser, 2007; Lange & Dewitte, 2019; Li et al., 2019; Steg & Vlek, 2009; Yuriev et al., 2020), and a single unifying theory has yet to be established. For the purposes of this chapter, we draw on the theory of planned behavior (Ajzen, 1985, 2002) because it is a social-cognitive model of behavior change that has been widely applied to understand how healthy behaviors within place settings might promote place attachment (Yuriev et al., 2020). The premise of the theory is that planned human behavior is precipitated by an intention to engage in a particular behavior (Davis et al., 2015). However, a person's intention to perform a behavior is shaped by a combination of antecedent influences (Godin et al., 2008; Norberg et al., 2007), including their attitude toward a particular behavior (e.g., a person's positive or negative evaluation of the behavior), subjective norms about the behavior (e.g., whether the behavior is considered socially acceptable), and their perceived control over being able to perform the behavior (e.g., how easy a person believes it is to engage in the behavior). Therefore, attitude, subjective norms, and perceived control are each theorized to affect planned behavior via their influence on behavioral intentions (Conner & Armitage, 1998; Yuriev et al., 2020). Together, the components that make up the theory of planned behavior highlight some of the antecedents of planned behaviors that may be relevant for building relationships with place.

As planned behaviors, pro-environmental behaviors refer to activities that people engage in to safeguard the environment and reduce the impact of environmental issues (e.g., climate change) on planetary health (Kollmuss & Agyeman, 2002; Yuriev et al., 2020). Pro-environmental behavior is a broad concept that could be reflected in a wide range of actions, such as participating in environmental activism, petitioning issues related to private and public spheres of environmentalism (e.g., saving energy, waste management), shifting to "green" modes of transportation (e.g., electric vehicles, cycling), or performing social behavior with the intention of promoting the welfare of individuals within an environment (Homburg & Stolberg, 2006; Muñoz et al., 2016; Ramus & Killmer, 2007).

In the aftermath of the COVID-19 pandemic and place attachment disruption that has unfolded, engagement in pro-environmental behavior will have roots in the social norms, attitudes of individuals, and the sense of perceived control that people have over engaging in pro-environmental behaviors. For example, in places where the burden of COVID-19 has been particularly high, the social norms concerning public engagement in pro-environmental behavior may deter a person from choosing to engage in pro-environmental behavior, even as the public health crisis wanes. In such instances, community leaders and local authorities may need to implement initiatives that reduce perceptions of risk and encourage people to interact with the broader environment, which could improve social norms about the value of participating in pro-environmental behavior. If the post-pandemic conditions within a particular context led to more positive attitudes, favorable social norms, and/or an increase in perceived control over participation in pro-environmental behavior, then the likelihood of people deciding to engage in pro-environmental behavior might increase. However, it is important to note that there could be numerous other factors that also affect whether people will engage in pro-environmental behaviors. Examples of factors that have the potential to either facilitate or thwart pro-environmental behavior include personal finances (e.g., availability of disposable income to engage in pro-environmental behavior) and physical capabilities (e.g., ability to perform certain activities within a place).

Pro-environmental behavior will vary based on the effort that is needed to engage in specific behaviors (Ramkissoon & Mavondo, 2014; Ramkissoon, Smith, et al., 2013; Ramkissoon, Weiler, et al., 2013). In the context of the COVID-19 pandemic, an example of a low effort pro-environmental behavior is signing an online petition against pandemic-related restrictions from the comfort of one's home. High effort pro-environmental behavior could include volunteering to be a part of the task force that implements physically demanding post-pandemic recovery initiatives within a city. As community mitigation strategies that have limited non-essential travel and in-person social interactions are gradually lifted, the effort that is required to engage in certain kinds of pro-environmental behavior is likely to diminish because the obstacles created by many of the public health measures would have been removed.

From Pro-environmental Behavior to Place Attachment

Regardless of the underlying reasons for engaging in pro-environmental behavior, research suggests that a person's bond with a particular place can be strengthened by behaviors (e.g., eco-friendly housing, community cleanups, planting trees) which serve to safeguard or improve environmental conditions (Scannell & Gifford, 2010b; Yuriev et al., 2020). Pro-environmental activities not only stimulate positive connections with places, but they can also bring people together (Boldero, 1995; Ramkissoon, 2020).

In Chapter 1, we introduced place attachment as the bond between a person and a place that is of significance to them. It is an overarching concept that comprises the affective (or place), behavioral (or person), and cognitive (or process) domains of attachment that can be developed with a particular place (Scannell & Gifford, 2010a). The place domain refers to the connections that people form with the natural and physical elements of the environment. The person domain entails how a person develops attachment to a place because of experiences, memories, and activities associated with that specific environment. The process domain emphasizes how people form attachment to the identity of a place by connecting with the culture and character of a particular place (see also Chapter 5).

Pro-environmental behaviors can intersect the different domains of place attachment. Existing research points to a positive association between place attachment and pro-environmental behavior (see Halpenny, 2010; Ramkissoon et al., 2012; Scannell & Gifford, 2010b; Zhang et al., 2014), but previous studies have largely relied on cross-sectional data that cannot be used to make inferences about causality. In the absence of clear evidence, the association between pro-environmental behavior and place attachment is likely bidirectional.

During the COVID-19 pandemic, many people have had their relationships with places of significance disrupted (Counted et al., 2021). Although there may be avenues to replace, compensate for, and recover from the resource loss that accompanies pandemic-related place attachment disruption (see Chapters 5, 6, and 7), people derive physical, psychological, and social benefits from forming and maintaining healthy bonds with places (Counted, 2019; Meagher & Cheadle, 2020; Rollero & De Piccoli, 2010; Scannell & Gifford, 2017). Hence, the post-pandemic recovery process should involve identifying and creating opportunities for people to re-establish or develop new relationships with places in the environment. We suggest that pro-environmental behavior could play a particularly useful role in facilitating connections with places that are in locations and settings that have either been inaccessible or have been avoided because of concerns about health and safety during the COVID-19 pandemic.

When considering the potential contributions of pro-environmental behavior to the post-pandemic recovery process, it is important to recognize that a person's engagement in pro-environmental behaviors could depend on the type, extent, intensity, and reparative processing of their pandemic-related place attachment disruption experience. For example, those within the first phase that could arise from place attachment disruption, protest, may be more likely to regain their place attachment by engaging in pro-environmental behaviors within the place they have been separated from. In the despair phase, people may be able to recover their attachment to a specific place that has been disrupted if their pro-environmental behavior within that place of attachment evolves incrementally and affords sufficient opportunity for them to successfully integrate their experience of place attachment disruption with their renewed relationship with that place. If the pro-environmental behavior that is initiated in a place of attachment that has been disrupted ends up triggering or aggravating the painful experience of separation distress, some people who are working through the despair phase may be unable to re-establish their lost bond with their place of attachment. However, people within the detachment phase may have relinquished their attachment to a former place of significance and may therefore be primed to use pro-environmental behavior to explore and develop a completely new attachment relationship.

Place Attachment and Flourishing

Attachment to a particular place (e.g., home, place of worship, neighborhood) can support well-being across a number of life domains. Studies have found that people who have healthy relationships with places tend to score higher on indicators of subjective well-being (e.g., life satisfaction), social well-being (e.g., social integration), physical health, mental health (e.g., lower anxiety), eudaimonic well-being (e.g., purpose in life), and overall quality of life (see Billig et al., 2006; Counted, 2019; Meagher & Cheadle, 2020; Rollero & De Piccoli, 2010; Tartaglia, 2013; Vada et al., 2019). The wide-ranging benefits that accompany place attachment resonate with the notion of individual human flourishing, which refers to "a state in which all aspects of a person's life are good" (VanderWeele, 2017, p. 8149).

Individual flourishing unfolds in a broader social, cultural, and environmental context (Rasmussen, 1999). Throughout human history, individual and collective experiences have transpired in places and spaces within the environment. Physical places have provided the backdrop for reaching meaningful milestones (e.g., a child's first steps), forming memories, bonding with others, and connecting with God or the divine. All of human life itself is inextricably connected to *place*. Although place is a constant feature in our everyday lives, the omnipresence of place often desensitizes us to the role that it plays in our pursuit of the highest ideals in life. If we are to understand what it means for individuals, communities, societies, and the natural environment of the earth to fully flourish as a collective, the concept of flourishing ought to address the notion that human life necessarily unfolds within the context of places. In recognition of this, we introduce the concept of *place flourishing* to capture the spectrum of flourishing layers, ranging from individual to planetary flourishing, that are bound together by the centrality of place in human life.

Just like individual flourishing is shaped by personal (e.g., education, family) and contextual (e.g., economic equality, religious liberty) dynamics (Keyes & Annas, 2009; VanderWeele, 2017), people who are flourishing (or languishing) will also have an influence on the well-being of their family members, friends, colleagues, and communities (Chambers et al., 2014; Prilleltensky & Prilleltensky, 2007). Hence, individual flourishing could have downstream implications for flourishing at other ecosystemic levels within society, the effects of which are likely to be complex and will vary based on the proximity of a person to a particular layer of flourishing within the wider ecosystem. For example, individual flourishing will have a stronger influence on layers of flourishing within society that are more proximal (e.g., one's own family) versus those that are more distal (e.g., the environmental health of the earth as a whole) to a person. Much empirical work is needed to identify and comprehensively understand the processes by which people-place relationships that develop from pro-environmental behavior might shape different layers of flourishing. In this chapter, we present an initial guiding framework that addresses pro-environmental behavior, place attachment, and place flourishing (see Fig. 8.1).

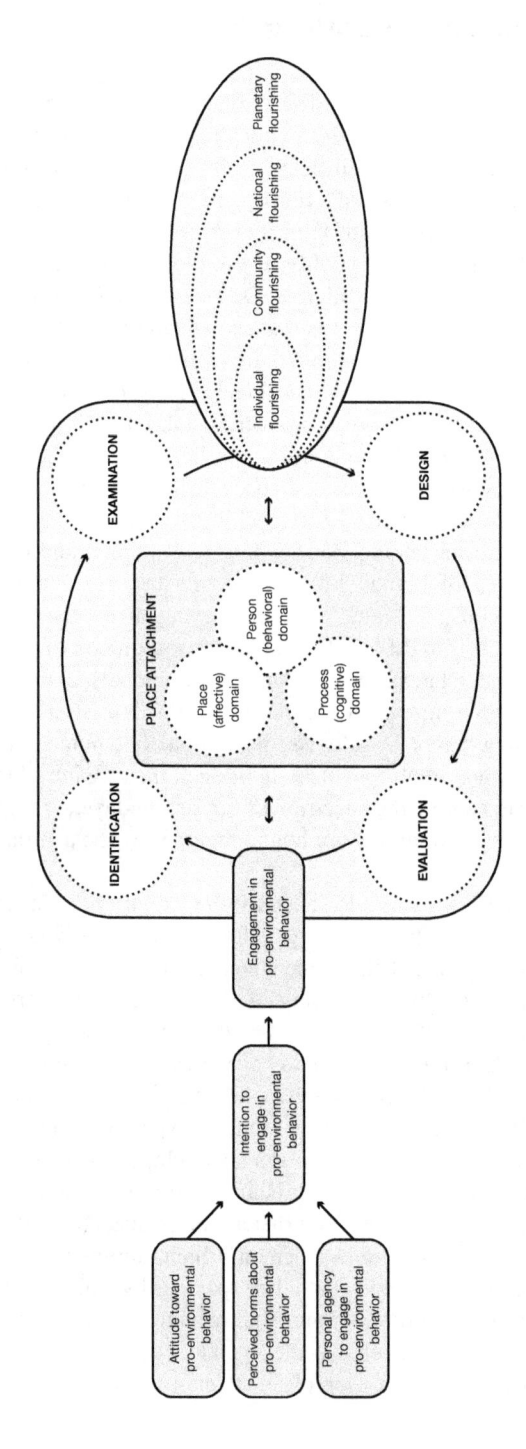

Fig. 8.1 Framework of place flourishing

Fostering Place Flourishing After a Pandemic

Having provided a brief overview of how pro-environmental behavior may enhance the well-being of individuals, communities, societies, and the planet by cultivating place attachment, we present an integrative framework that could be used to identify, understand, and encourage the kinds of pro-environmental behaviors that might lead to post-pandemic flourishing. Prior research suggests that pro-environmental behavior can be promoted by *identifying* which behaviors need to be changed to improve the quality of the environment, *examining* the determinants of those behaviors, *designing* and implementing interventions to modify targeted behaviors and their determinants, and *evaluating* the effectiveness of the interventions on the behaviors of interest, their determinants, and the quality of the environment and human life (Steg & Vlek, 2009). Together, these components reflect the pillars of Identification (I), Examination (E), Design (D), and Evaluation (E) that comprise the IEDE framework. Although the IEDE framework has been applied extensively to the promotion of pro-environmental behavior in general (see Steg et al., 2014; Steg & Vlek, 2009), we extend its application by considering its potential implications for encouraging the kinds of pro-environmental behaviors that might foster post-pandemic place attachment and flourishing. Figure 8.1 depicts how pro-environmental behavior may be involved in shaping place attachment processes, the implications of which could lead to higher levels of flourishing that begins at the individual level and extends through to the planetary level.

Identification

Encouraging people to engage in pro-environmental behavior that culminates in place flourishing will need to begin with an initial process of identifying post-pandemic activities (e.g., behaviors) that can be enacted to address the needs of the environment. This will require a two-part process. Given the environmental challenges that face our society (e.g., climate change), the first part involves identifying current behaviors that have a negative impact on the environment. For example, some human activities (e.g., deforestation) have altered environmental ecosystems in ways that increase the risk of natural disasters (O'Connor & Assaker, 2021). The second part entails identifying specific behaviors that are beneficial to the environment. For example, planting trees in local communities and reducing greenhouse gas emissions could have a positive impact on climate change (Domke et al., 2020). Context-specific inventories of behaviors that support or degrade environmental sustainability are likely to provide important foundational information that is needed to build pro-environmental interventions that support flourishing at different levels of society.

Examination

The second phase in fostering pro-environmental behaviors toward flourishing is the examination of social, cultural, and contextual factors (e.g., gender, religion, socioeconomic status) that might affect preferences and decisions about pro-environmental behavior. Such examination would need to begin with a feasibility assessment to identify the kinds of pro-environmental behaviors that are appropriate and can be realistically achieved by people within a particular context. Given the enormous economic impact that the COVID-19 pandemic has had on society, many people may be limited in their financial capacities to engage in some specific pro-environmental activities. It may be more reasonable to mobilize people to participate in community cleanups than it would be to ask people to travel long distances to support natural heritage areas that have been affected by the global economic slowdown. Although one of the purposes of encouraging pro-environmental behavior is to create awareness and increase people's engagement with the broader environment, not everyone will be interested in exploring new and unfamiliar environments after the COVID-19 pandemic (Majeed & Ramkissoon, 2020). It is possible that the residual effects of emplacement and social distancing will deter people from wanting to engage in high effort pro-environmental behavior.

Design

Once relevant pro-environmental behaviors and contextual factors that could affect the likelihood of those behaviors have been identified and examined, the next phase of the IEDE process involves designing customized interventions that aim to foster pro-environmental behavior within a particular context (Steg & Vlek, 2009). This process could be supported by using action-oriented methods in which a prototype intervention is designed alongside the community and then refined through feedback that is received from the community (Pfefferbaum et al., 2015). Action-oriented methods may need to be supplemented by other data collection techniques and sources (e.g., document analysis) that collectively provide a more holistic account of whether the planned interventions are accommodating the needs of both the environment and the communities in which they will be implemented. However, action-oriented methods are useful for designing context-specific interventions that can lead to social change and better inform policy and practice (Small, 1995).

Designing coordinated pro-environmental behavior interventions that address both the environmental needs and context-specific dynamics of individual people, communities, and nations is a complex and challenging endeavor. During the design phase, it may be useful to identify and align intervention objectives with international goals that center on achieving sustainable health and well-being for humanity. For example, the United Nations proposed a set of 17 interlinked Sustainable

Development Goals (SDGs) to promote a more sustainable future (do Paço & Laurett, 2019). Several of the SDGs address environmental issues that could inform decisions about which pro-environmental behaviors should be prioritized and targeted, including goals 6 (clean water and sanitation), 11 (sustainable cities and communities), and 15 (life on land). Implementing pro-environmental behavior interventions that align with relevant SDGs will require appropriate informational strategies (Steg & Vlek, 2009), such as setting up forums for engaging with communities and understanding the needs of local people. In addition to informational strategies, the design phase will also benefit from structural strategies that make the desired pro-environmental behavior more attractive or increase opportunities for people to engage in targeted behaviors. For example, reward systems could be implemented to increase engagement in desired pro-environmental behavior. If the interventions that are initiated to encourage pro-environmental behaviors are to be successful at fostering place attachment and ultimately flourishing, they need to sufficiently accommodate the contextual factors that could affect the effectiveness of those endeavors.

Evaluation

To identify the most practical and efficient use of resources for encouraging pro-environmental behaviors, the effectiveness of targeted approaches needs to be assessed and monitored (Ramkissoon, 2020). This process will involve generating data that can be used to guide immediate and future post-pandemic strategic planning. Assessing the effectiveness of pro-environmental behavioral interventions will require a focus on four primary areas. First, tracking changes in the determinants of pro-environmental behaviors will be important for identifying whether approaches that are used to encourage desired behaviors need to be modified over time. Second, changes in targeted behaviors need to be measured and monitored. Robust research is needed to gather high quality evidence on the effectiveness of strategies in changing pro-environmental behaviors. Third, changes in the needs and quality of the environment need to be assessed (Steg & Vlek, 2009). This entails evaluating the effectiveness of any new infrastructure that has been built to encourage and facilitate pro-environmental behaviors. Fourth, the evaluation process should include an assessment of changes in downstream outcomes of interest (e.g., place attachment, different layers of flourishing). Although this last component may be of particular interest to community leaders, public health experts, and policymakers, all four aspects of the evaluation phase are critical and will collectively contribute to ensuring that pro-environmental behaviors strengthen people-place relationships and support place flourishing.

Implications for Theory, Research, Policy, and Practice

We offer Fig. 8.1 as an initial framework that captures the potential for pro-environmental behavior to form part of initiatives aimed at facilitating post-pandemic flourishing. Although the framework is far from exhaustive and refinements will be necessary to enhance it, we encourage researchers, healthcare practitioners, and policy makers who are involved in post-pandemic recovery work to consider, expand upon, and integrate it into the initiatives they are undertaking to support the well-being of individuals, society, and the broader environment. Using this framework, we discuss some of the ways that theory, research, policy, and practice could contribute to achieving a common objective of sustainable post-pandemic place flourishing.

Theory

Many strides have been made toward understanding the nature, determinants, mechanisms, and outcomes associated with different types of flourishing (e.g., individual, community, planetary). However, considerable work remains to bring layers of flourishing together to form a more unified theoretical framework to guide the next wave of research, policy, and practice. In the process of providing a possible roadmap to fostering people-place relationships after the COVID-19 pandemic through targeting pro-environmental behavior, we discussed place flourishing as a way of capturing the idea that the highest form of well-being can be understood as a network of flourishing layers that are connected by the common underlying thread of *place*. It is an integrative approach to well-being because it brings together various layers of flourishing that extend from the smallest units of human life (e.g., the individual) through to the biggest (e.g., the planet). Although we recognize that our delineation of place flourishing will benefit greatly from refinements that expand the breadth and depth of its application, it offers one conceptual model that could support coordinated and systematic multidisciplinary research efforts that are centered on a core objective. Place flourishing may also affect how key stakeholders (e.g., environmental health specialists, mental health professionals) synergistically prioritize and attempt to promote flourishing.

At a more micro-level, place flourishing was introduced as a downstream consequence of the effect that pro-environmental behavior could have on place attachment. Theory and some empirical evidence support the linkage between place attachment and flourishing that is implied in Fig. 8.1. However, much of the current evidence for this association exists at the individual flourishing layer (e.g., Rollero & De Piccoli, 2010; Scannell & Gifford, 2017). It is our hope that the umbrella concept of place flourishing will prompt scholars to reconsider and expand existing frameworks on place attachment and well-being by attending to the complex, multifaceted, and reciprocal ways in which place attachment may be associated with different layers of flourishing.

Research

Post-pandemic research that draws on the IEDE process will need to employ methodologies that provide the highest quality evidence about the effectiveness of those interventions for encouraging the kinds of pro-environmental behaviors that cultivate place attachment and subsequent flourishing. Randomized controlled trials are the gold standard for evaluating the effectiveness of an intervention and establishing evidence of causation (VanderWeele et al., 2016), but using such an approach in pro-environmental behavior research may not always be feasible. One option that could yield valuable insights into the effectiveness of a pro-environmental behavior intervention is a randomized encouragement design (West et al., 2008). When larger-scale evaluations of effectiveness are necessary (e.g., community level), a nonrandom treatment assignment design (e.g., multiple baseline design) could be used (Hawkins et al., 2007). If the potential benefits of different types of pro-environmental behaviors are not well known, other research designs that provide a reasonable approximation of causality (e.g., longitudinal observational studies with propensity score matching) may be of some use in determining whether specific behaviors could be targeted to influence outcomes of interest.

Robust research on the effectiveness of pro-environmental behavior interventions will need to make use of metrics that are sensitive to the extent of change anticipated. If larger-scale interventions are implemented, layered measurement approaches may be necessary to evaluate effectiveness at different levels of potential impact. For example, interventions that target entire communities will benefit from measurement of individual (e.g., place attachment, individual flourishing) and community-level metrics (e.g., water quality, community well-being) that correspond with the areas in which post-intervention changes are expected. Importantly, research that accompanies pro-environmental behavior interventions must gather evidence that supports the overall IEDE process and would likely require modifications to remain relevant and effective over time. Ideally, evidence that is acquired through research on any pro-environmental behavior intervention would need to align with community, national, and planetary objectives that are developed to track the quality of people-place relationships and flourishing at different levels of society. However, research emphases will likely depend on whether policies are developed and refined to prioritize people-place relationships and place flourishing. Engaging in multidisciplinary research collaborations to systematically address different layers of flourishing could lead to policy changes that have broader and more holistic implications for well-being.

Policy

Given the unprecedented impact that the COVID-19 pandemic has had on people-place relationships (Counted et al., 2021), policies that are backed by dedicated funding streams could support post-pandemic flourishing by addressing the people-place relationship dimension of human life. Environmental justice and sustainability have become important priorities in the policy agendas of many countries (e.g., United Kingdom), with a growing emphasis on how environmental policies can help reduce inequalities for those at the margins of society (Amann et al., 2014). The framework proposed in Fig. 8.1 offers one approach that could serve a dual purpose of tackling environmental issues through pro-environmental behavior and closing gaps concerning inequalities in well-being, particularly if attempts are made to formulate policies based on a multilayered conception of flourishing that is rooted in place. Academic research focused on place flourishing should be made accessible to the public by local and national bodies that create opportunities for knowledge transfer, practice implementation, and industry engagement. Policies that build on the notion of place flourishing could have important benefits for people who are vulnerable to the myriad consequences that often underlie place attachment disruption, both in the context of a global crisis like the COVID-19 pandemic and more generally (e.g., natural disasters). By illuminating place as part of the fabric of human life, our view is that the COVID-19 pandemic has provided an opportunity for policymakers at different levels within societies (e.g., cities, states, countries) to explore policy options that harness *place* to accelerate post-pandemic recovery and positively transform post-pandemic life on earth.

Practice

The effectiveness of post-pandemic recovery initiatives that target pro-environmental behavior will depend on the ability of practitioners who are involved in those efforts (e.g., environmental health officers, urban planners, local community council officers) to successfully implement appropriate intervention strategies. As illustrated in Fig. 8.1, the IEDE model offers guidance on how to design, implement, and monitor the effectiveness of pro-environmental behavior interventions. However, a useful extension of the IEDE framework is the integration of place attachment and place flourishing as downstream benefits of planned pro-environmental behavior. The expanded framework retains a core focus on pro-environmental behavior as a key outcome of interest, but it offers practitioners an opportunity to consider how pro-environmental behaviors that are targeted might culminate in benefits that extend well beyond the behavioral changes that are expected.

Embracing this broader framework also brings into awareness the potential value that coordinated pro-environmental behavior strategies among practitioners could have on different layers of place flourishing. Practitioners who work in different locations, settings, and roles are encouraged to collaborate closely and freely share resources (e.g., data) with one another to support different layers of flourishing. The COVID-19 pandemic has shown that bold health policies, swift decision-making, and coordinated action can lead to more effective public health responses that are beneficial to the local and international community. Practitioners within local communities may be able to achieve the same kind of success by adopting a collaborative, streamlined approach in which specialists who are involved in pro-environmental behavior interventions at different layers within societies work together to achieve common objectives. Practitioners would also do well to collaborate with a network of professionals in other fields and sectors (e.g., commercial business, medicine, mental health, politics) to reinforce pro-environmental behavior initiatives. Partnering with professionals who have complementary expertise that can support the implementation of pro-environmental behavior interventions could lead to desirable long-term changes in behavior that nurture place flourishing.

Conclusion

As society begins to shift its focus toward what life might look like after the COVID-19 pandemic, it is important that we find suitable approaches to accelerate recovery and provide people with opportunities to pursue and sustain human flourishing. To this end, we proposed an integrative framework that can be adopted by researchers, healthcare practitioners, and policy makers to promote pro-environmental behavior, place attachment, and post-pandemic flourishing. Although initiatives that target different areas of human life will be needed to comprehensively facilitate post-pandemic recovery, we suggest that pro-environmental behaviors could yield a multifaceted range of benefits for human and planetary well-being. With growing environmental concerns threatening the future of life on earth, efforts that center on the promotion of pro-environmental behaviors in the aftermath of the COVID-19 pandemic may lead to valuable changes in the collective behaviors of humanity that support the long-term flourishing of both people and the planet that we call home.

References

Ajzen, I. (1985). From intentions to actions: A theory of planned behavior. In J. Kuhl & J. Beckmann (Eds.), *Action control: From cognition to behavior* (pp. 11–39). Springer. https://doi.org/10.1007/978-3-642-69746-3_2

Ajzen, I. (2002). Perceived behavioral control, self-efficacy, locus of control, and the theory of planned behavior. *Journal of Applied Social Psychology, 32*(4), 665–683. https://doi.org/10.1111/j.1559-1816.2002.tb00236.x

Amann, M., Roehrich, J., Essig, M., & Harland, C. (2014). Driving sustainable supply chain management in the public sector: The importance of public procurement in the European Union. *Supply Chain Management, 19*(3), 351–366. https://doi.org/10.1108/SCM-12-2013-0447

Bamberg, S., & Möser, G. (2007). Twenty years after Hines, Hungerford, and Tomera: A new meta-analysis of psycho-social determinants of pro-environmental behaviour. *Journal of Environmental Psychology, 27*(1), 14–25. https://doi.org/10.1016/j.jenvp.2006.12.002

Billig, M., Kohn, R., & Levav, I. (2006). Anticipatory stress in the population facing forced removal from the Gaza Strip. *Journal of Nervous and Mental Disease, 194*(3), 195–200. https://doi.org/10.1097/01.nmd.0000202489.78194.8d

Boldero, J. (1995). The prediction of household recycling of newspapers: The role of attitudes, intentions, and situational factors. *Journal of Applied Social Psychology, 25*(5), 440–462. https://doi.org/10.1111/j.1559-1816.1995.tb01598.x

Chambers, J. C., Bradley, B. A., Brown, C. S., D'Antonio, C., Germino, M. J., Grace, J. B., Hardegree, S.P., Miller, R.F., & Pyke, D. A. (2014). Resilience to stress and disturbance, and resistance to Bromus tectorum L. invasion in cold desert shrublands of western North America. *Ecosystems, 17*(2), 360–375.

Conner, M., & Armitage, C. J. (1998). Extending the theory of planned behavior: A review and avenues for further research. *Journal of Applied Social Psychology, 28*(15), 1429–1464. https://doi.org/10.1111/j.1559-1816.1998.tb01685.x

Counted, V. (2019). Sense of place attitudes and quality of life outcomes among African residents in a multicultural Australian society. *Journal of Community Psychology, 47*(2), 338–355. https://doi.org/10.1002/jcop.22124

Counted, V., Neff, M. A., Captari, L. E., & Cowden, R. G. (2021). Transcending place attachment disruptions during a public health crisis: Spiritual struggles, resilience, and transformation. *Journal of Psychology and Christianity, 39*(4), 276–286.

Davis, R., Campbell, R., Hildon, Z., Hobbs, L., & Michie, S. (2015). Theories of behaviour and behaviour change across the social and behavioural sciences: A scoping review. *Health Psychology Review, 9*(3), 323–344. https://doi.org/10.1080/17437199.2014.941722

Di Marco, M., Baker, M. L., Daszak, P., De Barro, P., Eskew, E. A., Godde, C. M., Harwood, T. D., Herrero, M., Hoskins, A. J., Johnson, E., Karesh, W. B., Machalaba, C., Garcia, J. N., Paini, D., Pirzl, R., Smith, M. S., Zambrana-Torrelio, C., & Ferrier, S. (2020). Opinion: Sustainable development must account for pandemic risk. *Proceedings of the National Academy of Sciences, 117*(8), 3888. https://doi.org/10.1073/pnas.2001655117

do Paço, A., & Laurett, R. (2019). Environmental behaviour and sustainable development. In W. L. Filho (Ed.), *Encyclopedia of sustainability in higher education* (pp. 555–560). Springer. https://doi.org/10.1007/978-3-319-63951-2_14-1

Domke, G. M., Oswalt, S. N., Walters, B. F., & Morin, R. S. (2020). Tree planting has the potential to increase carbon sequestration capacity of forests in the United States. *Proceedings of the National Academy of Sciences, 117*(40), 24649–24651. https://doi.org/10.1073/pnas.2010840117

Godin, G., Bélanger-Gravel, A., Eccles, M., & Grimshaw, J. (2008). Healthcare professionals' intentions and behaviours: A systematic review of studies based on social cognitive theories. *Implementation Science, 3*, 36. https://doi.org/10.1186/1748-5908-3-36

Halpenny, E. A. (2010). Pro-environmental behaviours and park visitors: The effect of place attachment. *Journal of Environmental Psychology, 30*(4), 409–421. https://doi.org/10.1016/j.jenvp.2010.04.006

Hawkins, N. G., Sanson-Fisher, R. W., Shakeshaft, A., D'Este, C., & Green, L. W. (2007). The multiple baseline design for evaluating population-based research. *American Journal of Preventive Medicine, 33*(2), 162–168. https://doi.org/10.1016/j.amepre.2007.03.020

Homburg, A., & Stolberg, A. (2006). Explaining pro-environmental behavior with a cognitive theory of stress. *Journal of Environmental Psychology, 26*(1), 1–14. https://doi.org/10.1016/j.jenvp.2006.03.003

Keyes, C. L. M., & Annas, J. (2009). Feeling good and functioning well: Distinctive concepts in ancient philosophy and contemporary science. *The Journal of Positive Psychology, 4*(3), 197–201. https://doi.org/10.1080/17439760902844228

Kollmuss, A., & Agyeman, J. (2002). Mind the gap: Why do people act environmentally and what are the barriers to pro-environmental behavior? *Environmental Education Research, 8*(3), 239–260. https://doi.org/10.1080/13504620220145401

Lange, F., & Dewitte, S. (2019). Measuring pro-environmental behavior: Review and recommendations. *Journal of Environmental Psychology, 63*, 92–100. https://doi.org/10.1016/j.jenvp.2019.04.009

Li, D., Zhao, L., Ma, S., Shao, S., & Zhang, L. (2019). What influences an individual's pro-environmental behavior? A literature review. *Resources, Conservation and Recycling, 146*, 28–34. https://doi.org/10.1016/j.resconrec.2019.03.024

Majeed, S., & Ramkissoon, H. (2020). Health, wellness, and place attachment during and post health pandemics. *Frontiers in Psychology, 11*, 573220. https://doi.org/10.3389/fpsyg.2020.573220

Meagher, B. R., & Cheadle, A. D. (2020). Distant from others, but close to home: The relationship between home attachment and mental health during COVID-19. *Journal of Environmental Psychology, 72*, 101516. https://doi.org/10.1016/j.jenvp.2020.101516

Muñoz, B., Monzon, A., & López, E. (2016). Transition to a cyclable city: Latent variables affecting bicycle commuting. *Transportation Research Part A: Policy and Practice, 84*, 4–17. https://doi.org/10.1016/j.tra.2015.10.006

Norberg, P. A., Horne, D. R., & Horne, D. A. (2007). The privacy paradox: Personal information disclosure intentions versus behaviors. *Journal of Consumer Affairs, 41*(1), 100–126. https://doi.org/10.1111/j.1745-6606.2006.00070.x

O'Connor, P., & Assaker, G. (2021). COVID-19's effects on future pro-environmental traveler behavior: An empirical examination using norm activation, economic sacrifices, and risk perception theories. *Journal of Sustainable Tourism*. Advance online publication. https://doi.org/10.1080/09669582.2021.1879821

Pfefferbaum, B., Pfefferbaum, R. L., & Van Horn, R. L. (2015). Community resilience interventions: Participatory, assessment-based, action-oriented processes. *American Behavioral Scientist, 59*(2), 238–253. https://doi.org/10.1177/0002764214550298

Prilleltensky, I., & Prilleltensky, O. (2007). Webs of well-being: The interdependence of personal, relational, organizational and communal well-being. In J. Haworth & G. Hart (Eds.), *Well-being: Individual, community and social perspectives* (pp. 57–74). Palgrave Macmillan. https://doi.org/10.1057/9780230287624_4

Ramkissoon, H. (2020). Perceived social impacts of tourism and quality-of-life: A new conceptual model. *Journal of Sustainable Tourism*. Advance online publication. https://doi.org/10.1080/09669582.2020.1858091

Ramkissoon, H., & Mavondo, F. (2014). Pro-environmental behavior: The link between place attachment and place satisfaction. *Tourism Analysis, 19*(6), 673–688. https://doi.org/10.3727/108354214X14146846679286

Ramkissoon, H., Smith, L. D. G., & Weiler, B. (2013). Testing the dimensionality of place attachment and its relationships with place satisfaction and pro-environmental behaviours: A structural equation modelling approach. *Tourism Management, 36*, 552–566. https://doi.org/10.1016/j.tourman.2012.09.003

Ramkissoon, H., Weiler, B., & Smith, L. D. G. (2012). Place attachment and pro-environmental behaviour in national parks: The development of a conceptual framework. *Journal of Sustainable Tourism, 20*(2), 257–276. https://doi.org/10.1080/09669582.2011.602194

Ramkissoon, H., Weiler, B., & Smith, L. D. G. (2013). Place attachment, place satisfaction and pro-environmental behaviour: A comparative assessment of multiple regression and structural equation modelling. *Journal of Policy Research in Tourism, Leisure and Events, 5*(3), 215–232. https://doi.org/10.1080/19407963.2013.776371

Ramus, C. A., & Killmer, A. B. C. (2007). Corporate greening through prosocial extrarole behaviours—A conceptual framework for employee motivation. *Business Strategy and the Environment, 16*(8), 554–570. https://doi.org/10.1002/bse.504

Rasmussen, D. B. (1999). Human flourishing and the appeal to human nature. *Social Philosophy and Policy, 16*(1), 1–43. https://doi.org/10.1017/S0265052500002235

Reese, G., Hamann, K. R. S., Heidbreder, L. M., Loy, L. S., Menzel, C., Neubert, S., Tröger, J., & Wullenkord, M. C. (2020). SARS-Cov-2 and environmental protection: A collective psychology agenda for environmental psychology research. *Journal of Environmental Psychology, 70*, 101444. https://doi.org/10.1016/j.jenvp.2020.101444

Rollero, C., & De Piccoli, N. (2010). Does place attachment affect social well-being? *European Review of Applied Psychology, 60*(4), 233–238. https://doi.org/10.1016/j.erap.2010.05.001

Scannell, L., & Gifford, R. (2010a). Defining place attachment: A tripartite organizing framework. *Journal of Environmental Psychology, 30*(1), 1–10. https://doi.org/10.1016/j.jenvp.2009.09.006

Scannell, L., & Gifford, R. (2010b). The relations between natural and civic place attachment and pro-environmental behavior. *Journal of Environmental Psychology, 30*(3), 289–297. https://doi.org/10.1016/j.jenvp.2010.01.010

Scannell, L., & Gifford, R. (2017). The experienced psychological benefits of place attachment. *Journal of Environmental Psychology, 51*, 256–269. https://doi.org/10.1016/j.jenvp.2017.04.001

Small, S. (1995). Action-oriented research: Models and methods. *Journal of Marriage and Family, 57*(4), 941–955. https://doi.org/10.2307/353414

Steg, L., Bolderdijk, J. W., Keizer, K., & Perlaviciute, G. (2014). An integrated framework for encouraging pro-environmental behaviour: The role of values, situational factors and goals. *Journal of Environmental Psychology, 38*, 104–115. https://doi.org/10.1016/j.jenvp.2014.01.002

Steg, L., & Vlek, C. (2009). Encouraging pro-environmental behaviour: An integrative review and research agenda. *Journal of Environmental Psychology, 29*(3), 309–317. https://doi.org/10.1016/j.jenvp.2008.10.004

Tartaglia, S. (2013). Different predictors of quality of life in urban environment. *Social Indicators Research, 113*(3), 1045–1053. https://doi.org/10.1007/s11205-012-0126-5

Vada, S., Prentice, C., & Hsiao, A. (2019). The influence of tourism experience and well-being on place attachment. *Journal of Retailing and Consumer Services, 47*, 322–330. https://doi.org/10.1016/j.jretconser.2018.12.007

VanderWeele, T. J. (2017). On the promotion of human flourishing. *Proceedings of the National Academy of Sciences, 114*(31), 8148–8156. https://doi.org/10.1073/pnas.1702996114

VanderWeele, T. J., Jackson, J. W., & Li, S. (2016). Causal inference and longitudinal data: A case study of religion and mental health. *Social Psychiatry and Psychiatric Epidemiology, 51*(11), 1457–1466. https://doi.org/10.1007/s00127-016-1281-9

West, S. G., Duan, N., Pequegnat, W., Gaist, P., Des Jarlais, D. C., Holtgrave, D., Szapocznik, J., Fishbein, M., Rapkin, B., Clatts, M., & Mullen, P. D. (2008). Alternatives to the randomized controlled trial. *American Journal of Public Health, 98*(8), 1359–1366. https://doi.org/10.2105/AJPH.2007.124446

Yuriev, A., Dahmen, M., Paillé, P., Boiral, O., & Guillaumie, L. (2020). Pro-environmental behaviors through the lens of the theory of planned behavior: A scoping review. *Resources, Conservation and Recycling, 155*, 104660. https://doi.org/10.1016/j.resconrec.2019.104660

Zhang, Y., Zhang, H. L., Zhang, J., & Cheng, S. (2014). Predicting residents' pro-environmental behaviors at tourist sites: The role of awareness of disaster's consequences, values, and place attachment. *Journal of Environmental Psychology, 40*, 131–146. https://doi.org/10.1016/j.jenvp.2014.06.001

Index

A
Action-oriented methods, 100
Attachment behavioral system, 2, 37
Attachment objects, 2
Attachment theory, 2–3, 37

B
Behavioral expressions, 56
Border resources, 42
Buddhism, 50

C
Cognitive-emotional processing, 83
Condition resources, 34, 40
Conservation of resources (COR) theory, 34–37, 41, 42
COVID-19 pandemic, 49, 51, 52, 55, 57, 59, 62, 63, 65, 66
   community-level aspects of life, 29
   dialectics of place, 4
      emplacement–displacement, 4, 5
      fixity–flow, 6
      inside–outside, 5, 6
   emplacement and displacement experiences, 15
   international health crisis, 1
   public health measures, 1
   relationships with place, 7
   scoping reviews on people–place relationships, 16, 28, 30

D
Despair, 55
Detachment, 55, 56, 64
Digital technologies, 29
Disrupted place attachment, 37
Distress, 47, 48

E
Emplacement, 5
Emplacement–displacement dialectic, 4, 5
Environmental psychology, 7

F
Fixities of place, 6
Fixity, 6

H
Hinduism, 47
Home attachment, 18, 20, 22

I
Identification, Examination, Design and Evaluation (IEDE) framework, 94
Inside–outside dialectic, 5

M
Mental health
   implications of home attachment, 20

© The Author(s), under exclusive license to Springer Nature Switzerland AG 2021
V. Counted et al., *Place and Post-Pandemic Flourishing*, SpringerBriefs in Psychology, https://doi.org/10.1007/978-3-030-82580-5

N
Nicomachean Ethics, 47

O
Object resources, 34, 37

P
Pandemic-related place attachment, 65
  place attachment disruption, 51
Pandemic resource ecology, 39, 42
People–place relationships, 1, 2, 16, 46
Personal resources, 34–36, 40, 41
Phenomenological attachment disruption, 56
Place attachment
  consequences, 47
  COVID-19 deaths, 45
  disruptions, 47, 49–51
  domains, 3
    person, 3
    place, 3
    process, 4
  ecological contexts, 38
  environment, 46
  environmental psychology, 2
  functions, 46
  and human–environment interactions, 8
  with interpersonal attachment, 2
  lockdowns, 45
  mortality and healthcare systems, 45
  people–place relationships, 46
  place-based concepts, 46
  place functions, 2, 46
  scoping review, 16
    data extraction and synthesis, 18, 19
    implications for research and practice, 28
    literature search, 17
    PRISMA-ScR flow diagram, 19, 20
    screening and selection, 17
    study characteristics, 19, 21–26
  secure base, 3
  social dimension, 4
  social-structural disadvantage, 49
  suffering, 46
  and tourism, 27, 28
  and well-being, 7, 8, 20, 27
Place attachment disruption, 3, 8, 33, 58, 60, 66
  COVID-19 pandemic, 57–59, 61, 71
  despair phase, 57, 63
  detachment, 38
  domain, 59
  ecological framework, resource loss, 38
  ecological propositions, 41–42
  forms, 62
  health crisis, 60
  immigration and globalization forces, 58
  implementation, 71
  integrated resource theory, 71
  mobilizing religious/spiritual resources, 74–76
  protest, 57, 60
  psychological distress, 72
  religion/spirituality, 71
  reparative responses, 61
  resilience, 76, 77
  resource investment, 35
  and resource loss, 37–38, 73, 74
  stressors, 71
  types, 58
Place confinement, 15
Post-pandemic funding, 7
Post-pandemic recovery, 38
Preferred Reporting Items for Systematic Reviews and Meta-Analyses extension for Scoping Reviews (PRISMA-ScR), 19, 20
Pro-environmental behavior
  components, 99
  COVID-19 pandemic, 93
  cultivating place attachment, 99
  design, 99–101
  environment and human life, 99
  evaluation, 101
  examination, 100
  flourishing, 97
  identification, 99
  implications, 99
    framework, 102
    policy, 104
    practice, 104, 105
    research, 103
    theory, 102
  integrative framework, 99
  place attachment, 95–97
  place-based experiences, 93
  place flourishing, 98
  planned behavior, 94, 95
  principles, 94
Proximity-seeking behavior, 37
Psychospiritual processes, 51
Public health crisis, 1, 2, 4–7, 29, 51
  on human–environment interactions, 16
Public safety measures, 5

Index

R
Reparative process, 55
Resource investment, 35, 36, 42
Resource loss
    COR theory, 34–37, 41, 42
    domains, 34
    at organizational level, 39
    principles
        desperation, 36
        gain paradox, 36
        primacy of loss, 35
        resource investment, 35
Resource recovery, 35, 36, 38

S
Self-regulatory functions, 82
Self-regulatory mechanisms, 82
Separation distress, 3
Separation-induced agitation, 63, 64
Separation-induced depression, 64
Severe acute respiratory syndrome coronavirus 2 (SARS-CoV-2), 64
    infection, 62
    outbreak, 1
Spirituality, 87, 88
Stay-at-home orders, 15
Suffering, 46–48, 50
    buddhism, 50
    conception, 48, 49
    form, 49, 50
Sustainable Development Goals (SDGs), 100–101

T
Tourism
    and place attachment, 27, 28
    virtual tools, 28
Transcending place attachment disruption, 64
    challenges, 83
    character strengths, 82, 83
    cognitive-emotional processing, 83
    COVID-19 pandemic, 82, 84
    gratitude, 84, 85
    health and well-being, 81
    hope, 85–87
    public health crisis, 81
    resource loss, 81
    spirituality, 87, 88
    virtues, 82, 83

V
Virtual experiences of places, 29

W
Well-being
    and place attachment, 20, 27

CPSIA information can be obtained
at www.ICGtesting.com
Printed in the USA
LVHW081918231121
704106LV00010B/66